Exoscope-Assisted Surgery in Otorhinolaryngology

Exoscope-Assisted Surgery in Otorhinolaryngology

Edited by

Armando De Virgilio, MD, PhD

Assistant Professor of Otorhinolaryngology-Head and Neck Surgery, Humanitas University, Milan, Italy

Giuseppe Spriano, MD

Professor and Chief of Otorhinolaryngology-Head and Neck Surgery, Humanitas University, Milan, Italy

ELSEVIER

Exoscope-Assisted Surgery in Otorhinolaryngology ISBN: 978-0-323-83168-0

Notices

Practitioners and researchers must always rely on their own experience and knowledge in evaluating and using any information, methods, compounds or experiments described herein. Because of rapid advances in the medical sciences, in particular, independent verification of diagnoses and drug dosages should be made. To the fullest extent of the law, no responsibility is assumed by Elsevier, authors, editors or contributors for any injury and/or damage to persons or property as a matter of products liability, negligence or otherwise, or from any use or operation of any methods, products, instructions, or ideas contained in the material herein.

Publisher: Cathleen Sether
Acquisitions Editor: Jessica McCool
Editorial Project Manager: Barbara Makinster
Project Manager: Sreejith Viswanathan
Cover Designer: Alan Studholme

3251 Riverport Lane
St. Louis, Missouri 63043

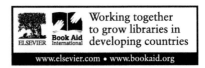

Contents

Contributors

Nicola Bisi, MD
Department of Otolaryngology, Head and Neck Surgery, University of Verona, Verona, Italy

Andrea Luigi Camillo Carobbio, MD
IRCCS Ospedale Policlinico San Martino, Genova, Italy; Department of Surgical Sciences and Integrated Diagnostics (DISC), University of Genoa, Genoa, Italy; Section of Otorhinolaryngology, Head and Neck Surgery – Azienda Ospedaliera di Padova, University of Padua, Padua, Italy

Filippo Carta, MD
Unit of Otorhinolaryngology, Department of Surgery, Azienda Ospedaliero-Universitaria di Cagliari, University of Cagliari, Cagliari, Italy

Giovanni Colombo, MD
Department of Biomedical Sciences, Humanitas University, Pieve Emanuele, Milan, Italy; Otorhinolaryngology Unit, IRCCS Humanitas Clinical and Research Center, Rozzano, Milan, Italy

Andrea Costantino, MD
Department of Biomedical Sciences, Humanitas University, Pieve Emanuele, Milan, Italy; Otorhinolaryngology Unit, IRCCS Humanitas Clinical and Research Center, Rozzano, Milan, Italy; Department of Otorhinolaryngology - Head and Neck Surgery, IRCCS Humanitas Research Hospital, Rozzano, Milan, Italy

Erika Crosetti, MD, PhD
Head and Neck Oncology Unit, Candiolo Cancer Institute, FPO – IRCCS, Candiolo, Turin, Italy

Giovanni Cugini, MD
Otorhinolaryngology Unit, IRCCS Humanitas Clinical and Research Center, Rozzano, Milan, Italy

Armando De Virgilio, MD, PhD
Assistant Professor of Otorhinolaryngology-Head and Neck Surgery, Humanitas University, Milan, Italy

Matteo Di Bari, MD
Department of Biomedical Sciences, Humanitas University, Pieve Emanuele, Milan, Italy; Otorhinolaryngology Unit, IRCCS Humanitas Clinical and Research Center, Rozzano, Milan, Italy

Davide Di Santo, MD
Otorhinolaryngology Unit, IRCCS Humanitas Clinical and Research Center, Rozzano, Milan, Italy

Fabio Ferreli, MD
Department of Biomedical Sciences, Humanitas University, Pieve Emanuele, Milan, Italy; Otorhinolaryngology Unit, IRCCS Humanitas Clinical and Research Center, Rozzano, Milan, Italy

Francesca Gaino, MD
Department of Otorhinolaryngology - Head and Neck Surgery, IRCCS Humanitas Research Hospital, Rozzano, Milan, Italy

Luca Malvezzi, MD
Department of Biomedical Sciences, Humanitas University, Pieve Emanuele, Milan, Italy; Otorhinolaryngology Unit, IRCCS Humanitas Clinical and Research Center, Rozzano, Milan, Italy

Daniele Marchioni, MD
Department of Otolaryngology, Head and Neck Surgery, University of Verona, Verona, Italy

Cinzia Mariani, MD
Unit of Otorhinolaryngology, Department of Surgery, Azienda Ospedaliero-Universitaria di Cagliari, University of Cagliari, Cagliari, Italy

Valeria Marrosu, MD
Unit of Otorhinolaryngology, Department of Surgery, Azienda Ospedaliero-Universitaria di Cagliari, University of Cagliari, Cagliari, Italy

Giuseppe Mercante, MD
Department of Biomedical Sciences, Humanitas University, Pieve Emanuele, Milan, Italy; Department of Otorhinolaryngology - Head and Neck Surgery, IRCCS Humanitas Research Hospital, Rozzano, Milan, Italy

Stefano Miceli, MD
Otorhinolaryngology Unit, IRCCS Humanitas Clinical and Research Center, Rozzano, Milan, Italy

Francesco Missale, MD
IRCCS Ospedale Policlinico San Martino, Genova, Italy; Department of Molecular and Translational Medicine, University of Brescia, Brescia, Italy

Gabriele Molteni, MD, PhD FEBORL-HNO
Department of Otolaryngology, Head and Neck Surgery, University of Verona, Verona, Italy

Giampiero Parrinello, MD
IRCCS Ospedale Policlinico San Martino, Genova, Italy

Giorgio Peretti, MD
IRCCS Ospedale Policlinico San Martino, Genova, Italy; Department of Surgical Sciences and Integrated Diagnostics (DISC), University of Genoa, Genoa, Italy

Francesca Pirola, MD
Department of Biomedical Sciences, Humanitas University, Pieve Emanuele, Milan, Italy; Otorhinolaryngology Unit, IRCCS Humanitas Clinical and Research Center, Rozzano, Milan, Italy

Roberto Puxeddu, MD, FRCS
Unit of Otorhinolaryngology, Department of Surgery, Azienda Ospedaliero-Universitaria di Cagliari, University of Cagliari, Cagliari, Italy

Vanessa Rossi, MD
Otorhinolaryngology Unit, IRCCS Humanitas Clinical and Research Center, Rozzano, Milan, Italy

Alessia Rubini, MD
Department of Otolaryngology, Head and Neck Surgery, University of Verona, Verona, Italy

Elena Russo, MD
Department of Biomedical Sciences, Humanitas University, Pieve Emanuele, Milan, Italy; Otorhinolaryngology Unit, IRCCS Humanitas Clinical and Research Center, Rozzano, Milan, Italy

Giuseppe Spriano, MD
Professor and Chief of Otorhinolaryngology-Head and Neck Surgery, Humanitas University, Milan, Italy

Giovanni Succo, MD, PhD
Head and Neck Oncology Unit, Candiolo Cancer Institute, FPO – IRCCS, Candiolo, Turin, Italy; Department of Oncology, University of Turin, Orbassano, Turin, Italy

Foreword

Minimally invasive surgery emerged in the 1980s as a safe and effective access technique for performing a surgical operation with less damage to the body than with traditional surgery. During the last 2 decades, most of the surgical community have come to prefer it to traditional (open) surgery, which requires larger incisions and usually a longer hospital stay. Since then, minimally invasive surgery has spread widely in many surgical specialties, such as general surgery, urogynecological surgery, and bariatric surgery, and lately, it has been revolutionized by advanced medical technology. In this regard, several new biomedical devices are continuously being introduced into clinical practice. The exoscopic technology was launched as an innovative tool carrying great visualization and magnification features. The operating exoscope provides a magnified three-dimensional (3D) view of the surgical field at various distances from the patient, allowing the surgeon to operate with precision, flexibility, and control, with a comfortable posture. The 3D view allows perception of depth of field to both first and assistant surgeons, thus becoming comparable to direct vision surgery. This technology may also provide educational and training opportunities for residents, fellows, students, and the operating room (OR) staff by permitting them to share with the surgeons the same vision of the surgical field through high-resolution 3D screens, in contrast to what occurs in 2D/microscope-based settings. As the surgical vision is shared, learners are able to understand procedures and gain confidence more quickly with the anatomic structures they will be dealing with. Beyond the advantage for teaching purposes, this can be crucial for increasing collaboration among the OR personnel resulting in an overall higher operating performance.

This textbook by A. De Virgilio and G. Spriano, the first dealing with this technology, is divided into sections offering a practical, clinically focused approach to the use of the 3D exoscope in the field of Otolaryngology and Head and Neck Surgery. Different surgical procedures, such as free flap reconstructive procedures, microlaryngeal surgery, lacrimal surgery, salivary glands surgery, and others are discussed in separate chapters. Technological principles are also addressed in detail. Moreover, a description of preclinical experiences performed in the clinical lab by students with the aim of comparing microscope and exoscope in first-time users is provided.

Exoscope-assisted surgery was recently introduced in clinical practice, thus only a few centers have long-lasting experience with this tool. It is the goal of this textbook to provide a comprehensive source of information regarding the advantages of exoscopic technology and its use in various surgical procedures. The authors of this book are experts in the field of Otolaryngology and Head and Neck Surgery and share their expertise and insights from years of collective experience in using the three-dimensional exoscope. The book should be of interest to anyone who is dealing with head and neck surgery, both physicians and allied health professionals.

Physician assistants and nurse practitioners who work with head and neck surgeons may also find this book valuable.

We should bear in mind that interactive teaching methods are of utmost importance to train globally minded healthcare professionals. We are hopeful that this comprehensive textbook on exoscopic technology from many experts in the field will provide readers with different perspectives on its clinical applications and future advances.

Marco Montorsi MD
Rector, Professor of Surgery
Humanitas University, Milan, Italy
President Emeritus Italian Society of Surgery

CHAPTER

Exoscopic technology

1

Armando De Virgilio, MD, PhD [1], **Andrea Costantino, MD** [2,3], **Elena Russo, MD** [2,3], **Vanessa Rossi, MD** [3], **Giuseppe Spriano, MD** [4]

[1]*Assistant Professor of Otorhinolaryngology-Head and Neck Surgery, Humanitas University, Milan, Italy;* [2]*Department of Biomedical Sciences, Humanitas University, Pieve Emanuele, Milan, Italy;* [3]*Otorhinolaryngology Unit, IRCCS Humanitas Clinical and Research Center, Rozzano, Milan, Italy;* [4]*Professor and Chief of Otorhinolaryngology-Head and Neck Surgery, Humanitas University, Milan, Italy*

1.1 Introduction

Microsurgical procedures have been developed during the last decades in several specialties. The operating microscope was indeed extensively used to perform fine and delicate surgeries in many fields. In particular, ENT surgeons usually perform ear, microlaryngeal, and skull base surgery with the operating microscope in daily surgical activity.[1–3] Moreover, head and neck free flap reconstruction is now widespread in many ENT centers.[4] The technological growth of the last decades have developed several instruments allowing for more precise surgery. In this context, exoscopic technology was introduced in the last decade as a new surgical visualization and magnification tool. The term "Exoscope" is derived from the Greek words "exō" (out of) + skopeîn (to look). In fact, the exoscope serves for observing and illuminating the surgical field from a position set apart from the patient's body. The surgeon could perform the microsurgical procedure by watching images on a screen thanks to advanced digital technology. Moreover, the novel three-dimensional exoscopes improved the hand and eye coordination allowing for the finest surgical maneuvers.

Several exoscopic devices have been developed during the last decade such as the VITOM (Karl Storz), Orbeye (Olympus), and Modus V (Synaptive Medical). Karl Storz's video telescope operating monitor (VITOM) was released in 2011, determining a change in direction for surgeries that used the traditional operating microscope. Several technical characteristics differentiate these devices such as illumination, magnification power, and the diameter of the field of view. Moreover, some important differences should be highlighted according to their portability other than from an economic perspective.

This chapter aims to provide a comprehensive analysis of technical characteristics of the exoscopic system to better understand its applicability in the various otolaryngology microsurgical procedures deeply explained in the following chapters.

Exoscope-Assisted Surgery in Otorhinolaryngology. https://doi.org/10.1016/B978-0-323-83168-0.00006-9

1.2 VITOM 2D

Around 2008, a new visualization system has been introduced in surgery in alternative to the operative microscope.[5] The high definition exoscope (HDXO-SCOPE) allowed to see the operating field from outside the body, in opposition to the endoscope in which the device is introduced into the body cavities. The telescope consisted in an autoclavable rigid lens (Fig. 1.1), which could be connected with a fiber optic light source (Xenon Nova 300; Karl Storz).

The telescope was characterized by a 10-mm outer diameter and a shaft length of 14 cm, allowing for a mean focal distance of 200 mm with a depth of field of 12 mm. It provided a high-resolution image with minimal spherical aberrations or chromatic distortions and a wide viewing angle comparable to the operating microscope. The telescope was connected to a three-chip sterilizable high-definition (HD) digitized camera with optical zoom and focus features. A medical-grade 23-in. HD (2 million pixels) video monitor (NDS Surgical Imaging, San Jose, California) was used for video display and documentation. The telescope was held in position by a pneumatic endoscope holder (Point Setter; Mitaka Kohki Co, Tokyo, Japan) with a wide range of motion. The device allows for push-button rapid repositioning with minimal drift, similarly to the hydraulic counterbalance system of the operating microscope.[6] Since the first exoscope system was developed in a two-dimensional view, the major limit was the relative lack of stereopsis compared to the operating microscope, resulting in a lack of image depth on the screen. This had an important impact on the overall surgical outcomes. It rendered difficult an accurate manipulation of microsurgical instruments and the hand-eye coordination was reduced when operating using a two-dimensional image. Depth perception can be obtained even in a monocular view thanks to interposition, motion, familiar size, and proximity-luminance covariance of the surgical field, allowing the surgeon to orient himself during surgery. However, this may not be enough under high magnification, especially in microsurgery, which requires even a higher precision.

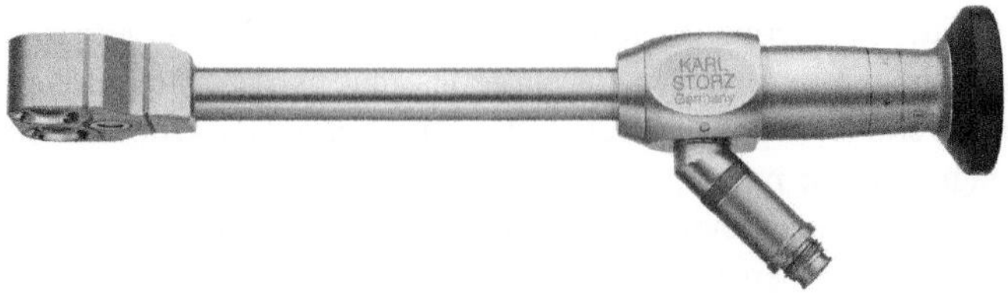

FIGURE 1.1

VITOM 2D telescope 90 degrees (Karl Storz, Tuttlingen, Germany).

1.3 Three-dimensional exoscopes introduction

The introduction of three-dimensional systems, which imply wearing dedicated glasses during surgery, mainly aimed to remedy the depth perception issue that characterized the 2D systems. The main advantage of three-dimensional exoscope systems is in fact the perception of objects' volume and the depth of structures for planning, targeting, and controlling fine movements, which was more difficult with two-dimensional visualization.[7]

This innovative and different approach to microsurgery encountered some resistance at first, as the adverse effects on the main operator were considerable in terms of visual strain, potential headache, and facial discomfort. Moreover, despite the higher image definition and the increased stereopsis, coordinating hand movements while looking at the screen was considered uncomfortable, especially compared to the operating microscope.

1.3.1 VITOM 3D

1.3.1.1 The camera

The VITOM 3D operating exoscope consists of a telescopic camera (Fig. 1.2) connected to a TV monitor system via IMAGE1 S platform (Fig. 1.3). This platform processes the image and displays it on the monitor in 4K resolution. The high resolution gives the surgical and operating room (OR) staff an extremely clear image of the surgical field.

The system's light source is from a table-top lighting system, feeding light to the surgical field via a fiber optic cable that fixes the camera. The power light-emitting diode (LED) 300 is a 300-W LED light that could be used to provide "cold light" to the surgical field (Fig. 1.4). However, other light sources such as the more powerful Xenon light from devices such as the XENON NOVA 300 could be used. The camera is connected to a control device (IMAGE1 PILOT) and has a magnifying power

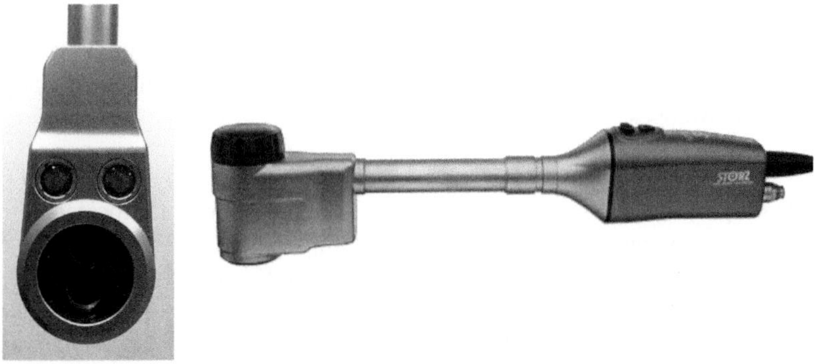

FIGURE 1.2

VITOM 3D with integrated illumination (Karl Storz, Tuttlingen, Germany).

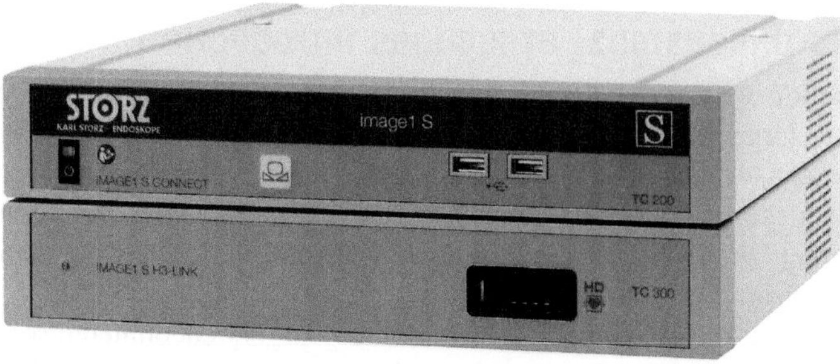

FIGURE 1.3

IMAGE1 S camera system (Karl Storz, Tuttlingen, Germany).

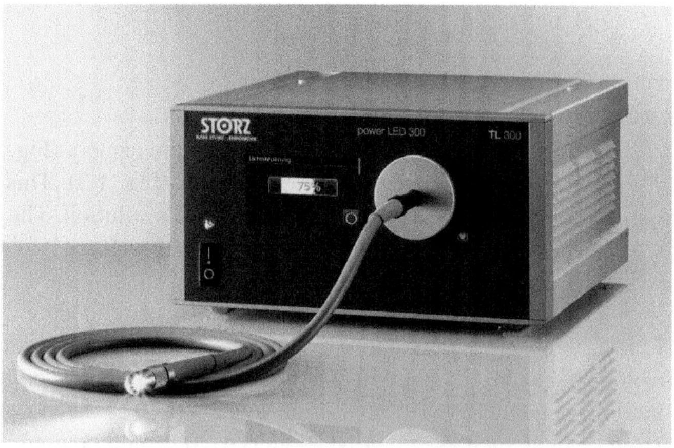

FIGURE 1.4

Cold light fountain POWER LED 300 SCB (Karl Storz, Tuttlingen, Germany).

of 8–30× and a depth of field of 7–44 mm. The VITOM's superior depth of field means that operators do not have to frequently adjust the focus, as they often do with operating microscopes.

1.3.1.2 The image

The VITOM projects the surgical image onto a 32-in. monitor that is located in front of the main surgeon, on the other side of the operating table (Fig. 1.5). This allows an optimal view for both the operator and other surgical staff without the interference of other OR members. Different from the operating microscope, the exoscope 3D camera does not have an adjustable telescopic lens. The magnified image on the monitor is just an enlarged view of the same image. Some operators claimed that there was a noticeable loss of image quality in the surgical field using older exoscope models.

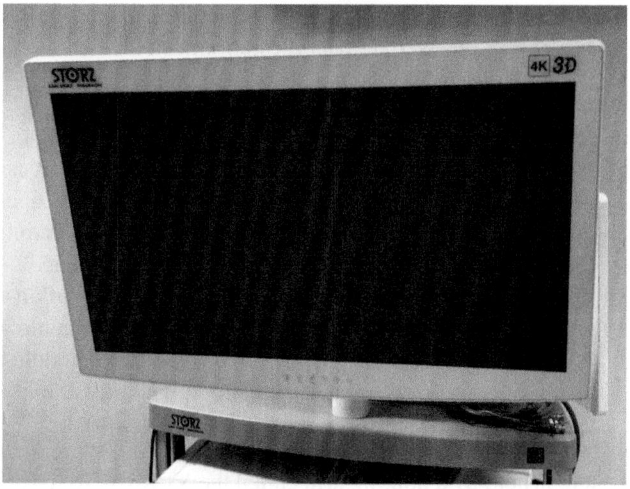

FIGURE 1.5

3D monitor (Karl Storz, Tuttlingen, Germany).

The new exoscopic systems project images at 4K resolution to overcome this issue, and the loss of resolution at zooming in may not affect the operator's ability to operate. The monitor is able to display the image in three dimensions (3D). Visualization in 3D requires the viewer to wear 3D glasses (Fig. 1.6). This 3D image allows the surgeon to have a better view of the surgical field as they can see with depth perception as well as in 4K resolution.

The exoscopic camera could be also combined to an endoscope thanks to the picture-in-picture display modality. In particular, the screen can show two different 2D images simultaneously to allow for a combined approach. This modality was

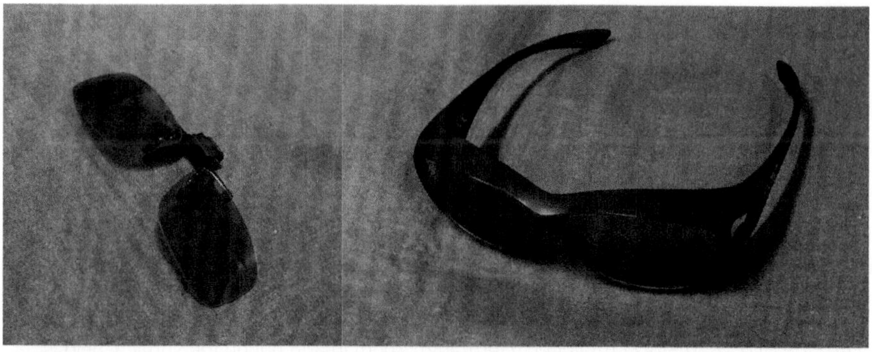

FIGURE 1.6

3D Polarization glasses (*right*) and 3D clip-on glasses (*left*) (Karl Storz, Tuttlingen, Germany).

proposed for lacrimal surgery to show the outer ocular field (exoscope) and the nasal cavity (endoscope) during endoscopic dacryocystorhinostomy.[8]

1.3.1.3 Control unit

The operating camera system is controlled by a specifically created device called IMAGE1 PILOT (Fig. 1.7). Owing to the compact size of the device, it can be placed around the operating bed and can be easily controlled by the second operator or the scrubbed nurse. The controller is essentially a joystick with an intuitive design. Limited prior experience is needed given the ease of use of this device in modifying the camera settings. The IMAGE1 PILOT is able to zoom in and out on the surgical field by pulling or pushing in the joystick. The focus of the camera could be modified by rotation of the joystick, while the image projected on the screen could be adjusted by moving up, down, left, and right on the joystick on the vertical axis (Fig. 1.7).

1.3.1.4 Holding system

The camera system is held by a holding arm called the VERSACRANE holding system (Fig. 1.8). The main advantage of this system is the smaller size and the greater maneuverability if compared to some of the larger operating microscopes. Many joints of this system can be manually adjusted by the operator to place the camera in many different positions. The holding system allows for a focal distance from 20 to 50 cm depending on the surgical procedures. Recently, the ARTip *cruise* robotic system (Fig. 1.9) was introduced by the Karl Storz company (Tuttlingen, Germany) to improve the maneuverability and the precision of the 3D camera.[2] The motorized holding arm leads to an intuitive and precise position of the camera with the opportunity to maintain a stable view. Moreover, a pivot movement around the focal point allows the surgeon to reach complex viewing angles with optimal accuracy. Setup of the system is easy and fast thanks to position presets, which memorize standard robotic arm positions. The ARTip *cruise* can be precisely moved to

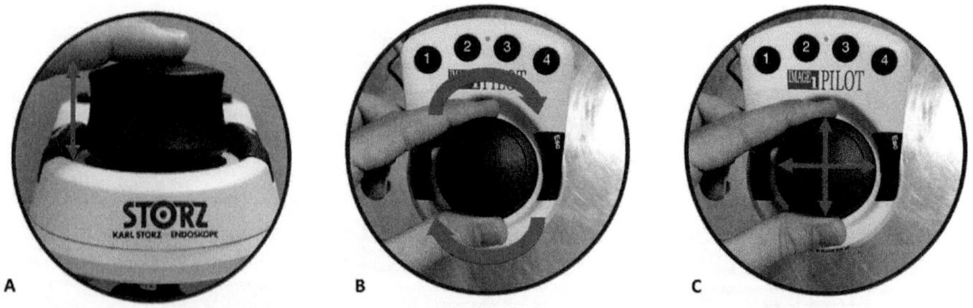

FIGURE 1.7

IMAGE1 PILOT (Karl Storz, Tuttlingen, Germany). Zoom in and out on the surgical field is performed by pulling or pushing in the joystick (A). The focus of the camera could be modified by the rotation of the joystick (B). The image projected on the screen could be adjusted by moving up, down, left, and right on the joystick (C).

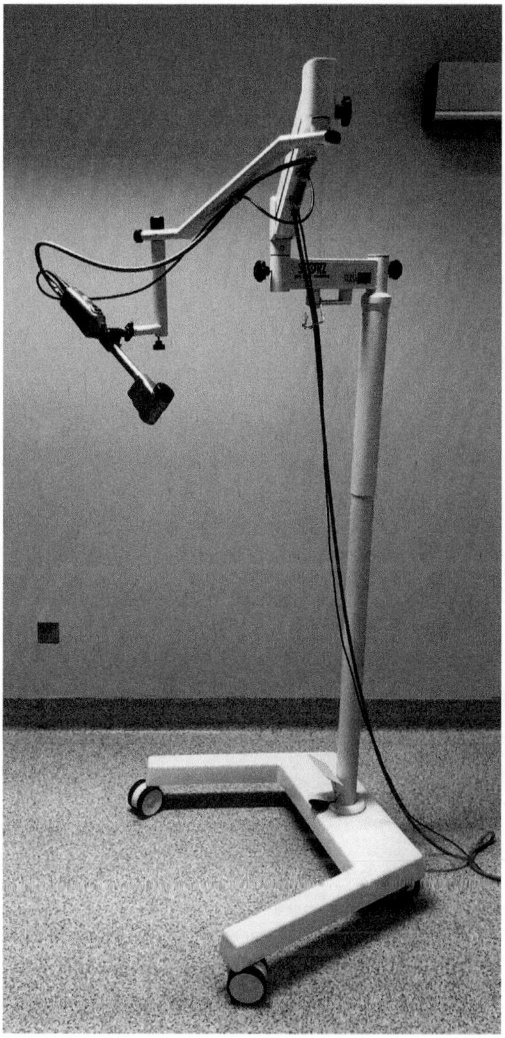

FIGURE 1.8

VERSACRANE holding system (Karl Storz, Tuttlingen, Germany).

control each degree of freedom individually (X, Y, Z, Pivot, Rotation) using only one hand that manipulates the IMAGE1 PILOT.

As a consequence, the surgeon has a free hand able to maintain surgical instruments during camera movements. A foot pedal can be used to switch between VITOM 3D and the ARTip *cruise* control with the IMAGE1 PILOT. However, this holding system is more cumbersome if compared to the VERSACRANE holding system, and further studies are needed to confirm its real benefit.[9]

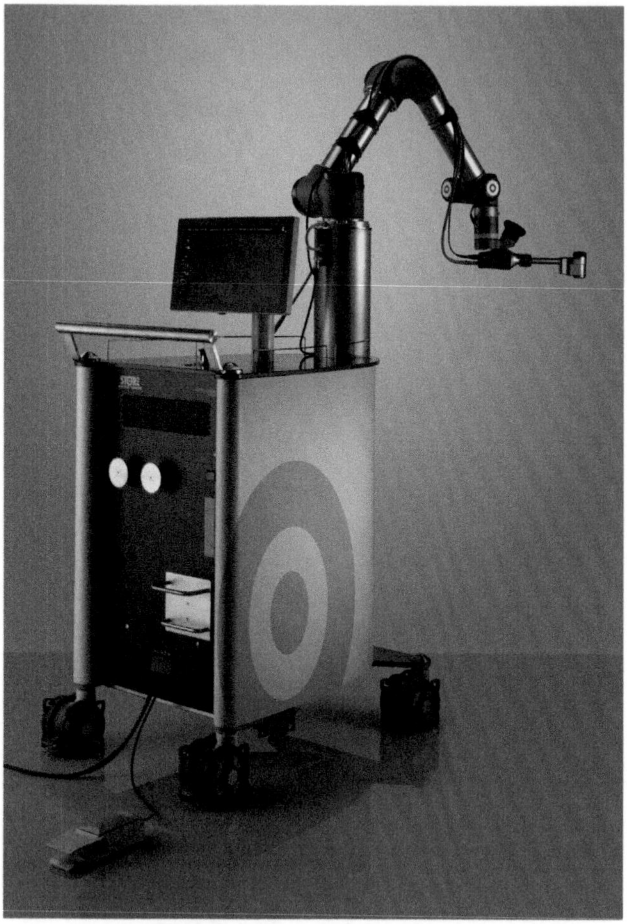

FIGURE 1.9

ARTip *cruise* robotic system (Karl Storz, Tuttlingen, Germany).

1.3.1.5 Set-up

Different surgical procedures could be performed with the aid of the exoscope, as mentioned earlier. Some differences in terms of OR set-up should be outlined to make the best use of the exoscopic technology. The small size of the 3D camera and the slim holding system allow for the placement of all the tools without any interferences with the surgical field. Each procedure needs the placement of the holding system and the screen in a specific position to ensure that the main surgeon, the scrub nurse, and any assistants to adequately perform surgery (see the following chapters for details). The vertical column equipped with the 32-in. monitor, the IMAGE1 S platform, and the light source should be placed in front of the main surgeon, given that the optimal 3D vision could be achieved only with the gaze perpendicular to the screen. The main screen is enough for both the main surgeon and scrub nurse in many surgical procedures (e.g., microlaryngeal surgery or free flap reconstruction). However, we should mention that an additional screen could be placed in front of the assistant and the scrub nurse if required by the OR setting. An example of surgical setting for microsurgical anastomosis is illustrated in Fig. 1.10.

1.3.1.6 Customisability and costs

The benefits of the VITOM system are the customisability and its ease of use. The system can be attached to different controllers, holders, light sources, and camera systems. For instance, the IMAGE1 S is compatible with cameras used in a variety of situations from laparoscopic surgeries to outpatient laryngoscopy. The user is free to modify the camera or attachments to suit their surgical needs and the available instruments in the center. As previously mentioned, the light source is interchangeable. If the procedure has a greater demand for luminosity, a Xenon light source could be used instead of an LED light source. This customisability allows the VITOM to be used in a myriad of surgeries as it can be adapted to surgical needs. As a consequence, the economic burden of this new technology could be balanced by the extensive use in various head and neck surgical procedures. Even more important is that some instruments used in exoscopic technology are derived from

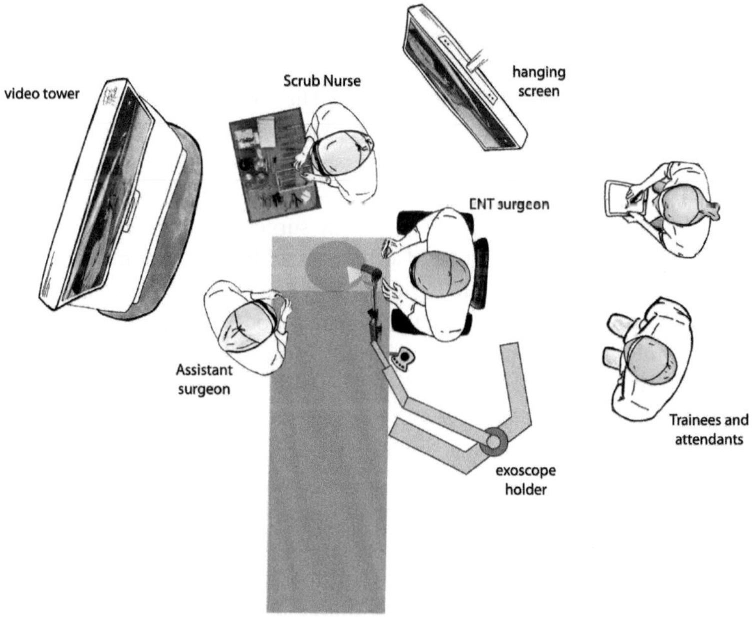

FIGURE 1.10

Surgical setting for microsurgical anastomosis. A second 3D screen can be used by the assistant surgeon.

endoscopic surgery. In particular, the 4K screen, the IMAGE1 S platform, and the light source that construct the endoscopic column are usually available in almost all ENT centers. As a consequence, the costs of the VITOM 3D exoscope are limited to 45,000 $ if we considered the specific instrument (3D exoscopic camera, holding system, and IMAGE1 PILOT) needed by this technology. Otherwise, the price of the VITOM system in the United States including various accessories is approximately 250,000 $. Although a direct comparison with the operating microscope could not be performed due to its wide range of prices, this system seems to present a favorable cost-benefit ratio that needs to be confirmed by further economic studies.

Finally, the possibility to easily record images of the surgical procedures thanks to the compatibility to the majority of recording systems represents a great advantage of this technology. It is possible to capture the camera's image or video in HD or 4K resolution as well as in 3D. The ability to capture video in such high definition is another advantage over the traditional operating microscope for educational purposes.

1.3.2 ORBEYE

The ORBEYE (Olympus, Tokyo, Japan) was launched in 2017 as a new 4K three-dimensional technology.[10]

The standalone optical system is based on semiconductor cameras with a very high resolution (3840 × 2160 pixels), supported by a semirobotic counterbalanced arm. Focusing and zooming could be controlled by hand at the scope unit or by the use of a footswitch. The focal length of the exoscope is 220–550 mm, while the field of view ranges from 7.5 to 171 mm. The total zoom function allows for a magnification change ratio from 1 to 12 (Optical 1:6, Digital 1:1.5 or 1:2) depending on the configuration. Polarization 3D glasses are required for proper viewing of the monitor images. The ORBEYE system is standardly associated with a greater screen (55 in.) that should be placed far from the surgeon to allow for a good vision. A secondary, smaller monitor can be also used in addition to the main one.

In addition to the standard white light imaging, the ORBEYE system offers three different visualization modes. An infrared imaging mode that provides bright 4K 3D intraoperative indocyanine green fluorescence to ensures brighter illumination of the vascular structures. ORBEYE uses dedicated LEDs capable of directly producing the required wave-length without relying on filter technology. A blue light imaging mode could be used to distinguish tissues that have accumulated specific fluorophores (5-aminolevulinic acid) thanks to a dedicated blue light LED. This technology provides high contrast and illumination to improve dissection precision. Finally, a narrow band imaging technology is provided to visualize the different vascular patterns of the tissues.

The price of the system in the United States including various accessories is approximately 450,000 $.

1.3.3 Modus V

The Modus V was released in 2017 by the Synaptive Medical Inc. company.[11] It is a digital exoscope with robotic arm technology based on the Canadarm device employed on the International Space Station. It incorporates a high-powered microscope, hands-free tracking of surgical instruments, automatic focus of the area of interest, preprogramming of procedural steps, and a wide range of robotic arm motion. Modus V has a 12.5× optical zoom, while the field of view ranges from 6.5 to 207.9 mm. A 3D visualization was recently introduced to overcome the limits against the other systems.

The price of the system in the United States including various accessories is approximately variable between 600,000 and 750,000 $.

1.4 Pearls and pitfalls

- Exoscopic technology was introduced in the last decade as a new surgical visualization and magnification tool to substitute the operating microscope.
- The surgeon could perform the microsurgical procedure by watching high-definition images on a flat screen thanks to advanced digital technology.
- The three-dimensional exoscopes improve hand and eye coordination allowing for the finest surgical maneuvers.
- Various exoscopic systems have some technical differences that should be considered during surgery.
- The operating room set-up is slightly different based on the microsurgical procedure performed.
- The VITOM 3D system can be attached to different controllers, holders, light sources, and camera systems and could be used in various head and neck surgical procedures reducing the economic burden.

References

1. Smith S, Kozin ED, Kanumuri VV, et al. Initial experience with 3-dimensional exoscope-assisted transmastoid and lateral skull base surgery. *Otolaryngol Head Neck Surg*. 2019; 160(2):364–367.
2. De Virgilio A, Costantino A, Mondello T, et al. Pre-Clinical experience with the VITOM 3D and the ARTip cruise system for micro-laryngeal surgery. *Laryngoscope*. 2021; 131(1):136–138.
3. Rubini A, Di Gioia S, Marchioni D. 3D exoscopic surgery of lateral skull base. *Eur Arch Otorhinolaryngol*. 2020;277(3):687–694.
4. De Virgilio A, Mercante G, Gaino F, et al. Preliminary clinical experience with the 4 K3-dimensional microvideoscope (VITOM 3D) system for free flap head and neck reconstruction. *Head Neck*. 2020;42(1):138–140.

5. Mamelak AN, Danielpour M, Black KL, Hagike M, Berci G. A high-definition exoscope system for neurosurgery and other microsurgical disciplines: preliminary report. *Surg Innov*. 2008;15(1):38–46.
6. Shirzadi A, Mukherjee D, Drazin DG, et al. Use of the video telescope operating monitor (VITOM) as an alternative to the operating microscope in spine surgery. *Spine*. 2012; 37(24):E1517–E1523.
7. Ricciardi L, Chaichana KL, Cardia A, et al. The exoscope in neurosurgery: an innovative "point of view". A systematic review of the technical, surgical and educational aspects. *World Neurosurg*. 2019. S1878–8750(19)30080-30084.
8. Pirola F, Spriano G, Malvezzi L. Preliminary experience with exoscope in lacrimal surgery. *Eur Arch Otorhinolaryngol*. 2020. https://doi.org/10.1007/s00405-020-06379-9.
9. De Virgilio A, Costantino A, Ebm C, et al. High definition three-dimensional exoscope (VITOM 3D) for microsurgery training: a preliminary experience. *Eur Arch Otorhinolaryngol*. 2020;277(9):2589–2595.
10. Takahashi S, Toda M, Nishimoto M, et al. Pros and cons of using ORBEYE™ for microneurosurgery. *Clin Neurol Neurosurg*. 2018;174:57–62.
11. Pafitanis G, Hadjiandreou M, Alamri A, Uff C, Walsh D, Myers S. The Exoscope versus operating microscope in microvascular surgery: a simulation non-inferiority trial. *Arch Plast Surg*. 2020;47(3):242–249.

CHAPTER 2

Educational role and preclinical application of exoscope-assisted surgery

Armando De Virgilio, MD, PhD [1], Andrea Costantino, MD [2,3], Elena Russo, MD [2,3], Stefano Miceli, MD [3], Francesca Pirola, MD [2,3], Giuseppe Spriano, MD [4]

[1]*Assistant Professor of Otorhinolaryngology-Head and Neck Surgery, Humanitas University, Milan, Italy;* [2]*Department of Biomedical Sciences, Humanitas University, Pieve Emanuele, Milan, Italy;* [3]*Otorhinolaryngology Unit, IRCCS Humanitas Clinical and Research Center, Rozzano, Milan, Italy;* [4]*Professor and Chief of Otorhinolaryngology-Head and Neck Surgery, Humanitas University, Milan, Italy*

2.1 Role and importance of education in microsurgery

Microsurgery was first introduced in the otolaryngology field at the beginning of the 900s.[1] In 1921, a monocular microscope with a high magnification was first used in ear surgery for the need of a surgical field magnification for the visualization of restricted areas. This introduction required proper training of surgeons to work in a different way, with a higher magnification and with a restricted view, as well as the development of specialized instruments that could allow proper tissue handling in a finer and more precise way. Microsurgical procedures are now widespread in many specialties, and surgical training has gained importance in this context.[2]

The American College of Surgeons—Accredited Education Institutes promote surgical simulation in the education and training of residents, and indeed, it represents an important requirement for accreditation of surgical residency programs in the United States.[3] Microvascular surgery is one of the most demanding operative technical skills in surgery, and the microsurgical training differs from other fields due to several factors. Different basic microsurgical skills, such as operating a microscope or using microsurgery instruments, are needed to adequately perform the various procedures. The refined movements and precision required in microsurgery make it technically challenging, and it is indeed associated with a very steep learning curve. Formal course in microsurgery is usually conducted before operating on patients. Simulation-based training is usually performed in a laboratory setting with microscopes and live animal subjects. Moreover, several nonliving models have been developed to expedite the microsurgical learning curve in a less expensive and more ethical setting.[4]

Exoscopic technology was introduced in the clinical practice to substitute the operating microscope, and various surgical procedures have been performed with optimistic clinical outcomes.[5–7] The possibility to improve the surgeons' skills in operating with the exoscope will have a great impact from this perspective. The

Exoscope-Assisted Surgery in Otorhinolaryngology. https://doi.org/10.1016/B978-0-323-83168-0.00007-0

advent of exoscope-based microsurgical training with surely expedite the widespread of this new technology, that may replace the operating microscope in many ENT centers in the near future.

2.2 Microsurgery training with exoscopic technology

The exoscope is a reliable tool for first-time users in the microsurgery training setting. As already mentioned, a simulation-based training is usually performed in a laboratory setting to improve the abilities in performing microsurgical tasks. During the last decades, the operating microscope was used to perform different kinds of microsurgical procedures in the preclinical setting. Given the widespread of the exoscopic technology in the clinical context, we expect that more and more courses will be organized to improve the ability of naïve surgeons before the clinical application.

Exoscope-based microsurgical training will gain importance for two main reasons. First, the exoscope represents a new technology, and a specific knowledge is needed to adequately use it. The operating room (OR) set-up is planned on the basis of the surgical procedure, and the surgeon should exactly know how to place the instruments (e.g., the holding system, the screen) to benefit from the exoscope ergonomics. Moreover, the surgeon should be able to manage any technological issues that could be encountered in the clinical setting. For example, the IMAGE1 PILOT should be connected to the IMAGE 1S platform when it is placed on a perfect horizontal plane. Otherwise, the image would not be fixed on the screen during the procedure, forcing the surgeon to repeatedly set the camera with longer procedure time and fragmented surgical steps. Second, the microsurgical procedures that could be performed with the exoscope are essentially unaffected by the surgical visualization and magnification tool used in terms of surgical steps. However, the surgeon should become accustomed to the new surgical visualization and magnification tool. In fact, the gaze is directed to the screen and not to the binocular microscope, and a different posture should be maintained during the surgery.

We performed a preclinical study in a simulation laboratory setting using the video telescope operating monitor (VITOM) 3D exoscope (Fig. 2.1). The study was divided into two phases. The first phase was designed to assess the feasibility of an exoscope-based microsurgical simulation. The second phase was designed to compare the exoscope and the operating microscope.

Basic microsurgical exercises were proposed to first-time users. In particular, a battery of four exercises related to different surgical procedures was tested to evaluate the feasibility and the quality of the surgical training with both systems. Objective and subjective parameters were analyzed for comparison. Advantages and disadvantages were also assessed through a self-reported subjective analysis.

2.2.1 Feasibility of exoscope-based training

Naïve medical students with no prior experience in microsurgery were chosen. Before perform the exercises, all students attended a lesson specifically prepared to show how the tasks should be performed. Moreover, the VITOM 3D exoscope

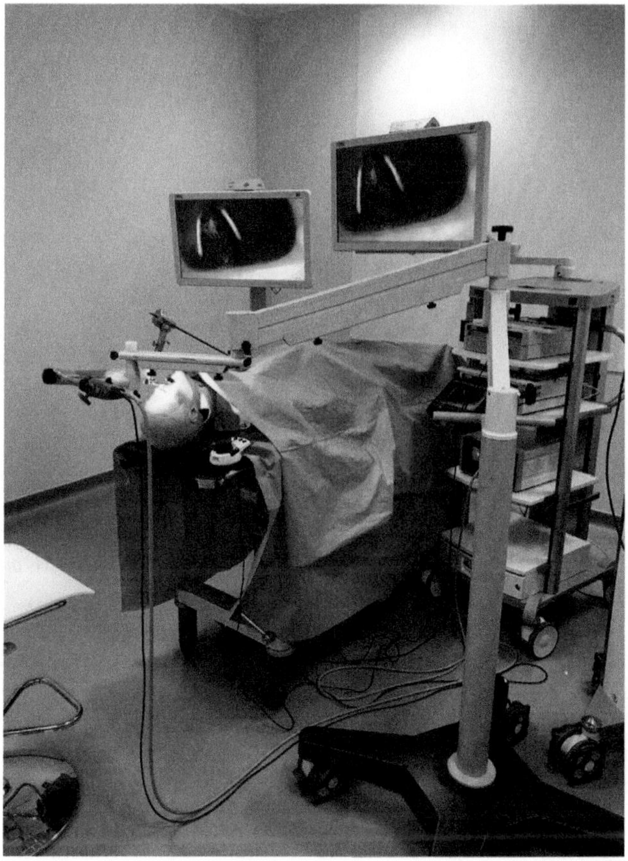

FIGURE 2.1

Simulation setting with the 3D VITOM 3D mounted on the VERSACRANE in the microlaryngeal test.

and the operating microscope (Zeiss OPMI CS NC31) general properties and the manipulation instructions were provided before starting the simulation. All students performed the following battery of four exercises able to assess basic microsurgical skills (Fig. 2.2):

- *Maneuvering test* (Fig. 2.2A): four different coins were placed on a blue hard surface to form a rhombus with the minor and major diagonals of 20 and 40 cm, respectively. The four coins were also placed at different heights to make the test more challenging. The student was instructed to move the exoscope or the microscope to focus all the coins in a specific sequence. A good vision of all coins should be obtained changing only the focal distance to conclude the task.
- *Gauze test* (Fig. 2.2B): a single sheet of gauze of known size was fixed on a flat surface, and the student was instructed to remove a single thread of the gauze. According to the gauze web-like structure, the students had to unthread a single "box" at once using microsurgery forceps. The length of the thread removed was measured after a fixed time of 2 min.

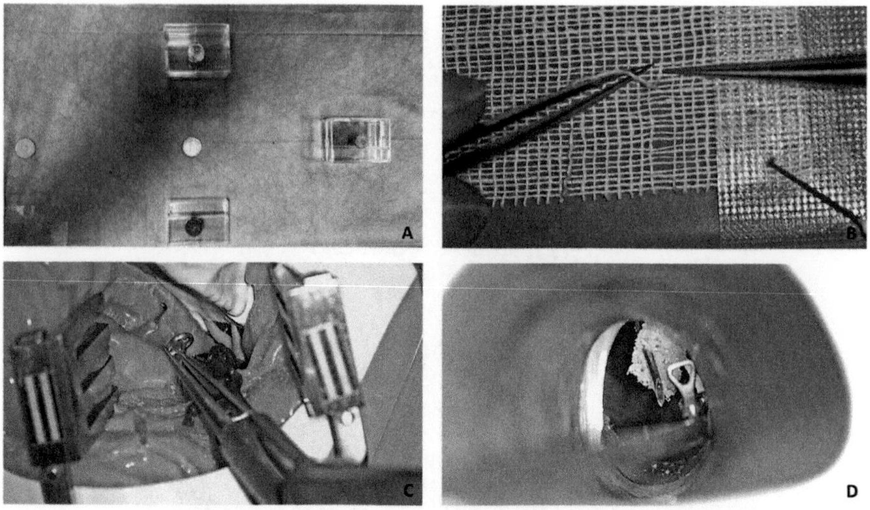

FIGURE 2.2

Microsurgical exercises performed with the VITOM 3D maneuvering test (A), gauze test (B), pterional model test (C), and microlaryngeal test (D).

- *Pterional model test* (Fig. 2.2C): Three different metal bars were placed inside the cerebral tissue of a pterional craniotomy model (*UpSim* by UpSurgeOn). In particular, the bars were placed at different depths related to the neurovascular structures to require a refocusing during the exercise. The students were instructed to put a metal circular ring over each bar using microsurgery forceps in a specific sequence.
- *Microlaryngeal test*[8] (Fig. 2.2D): A medium size-operating laryngoscope (Kleinsasser, Karl Storz, Tuttlingen, Germany) was used to visualize the vocal cords of a human-size silicon mannequin placed in the Boyce position. A small size needle (13 mm, 30G) was fixed at the level of anterior commissure. The student was instructed to focus on the glottis plane, and to insert, leave, and take it back a small (3 mm diameter) piece of cottonoid on the needle. The exercise was performed using microlaryngeal grasping forceps.

The majority of studies involving microsurgery training include knot tying and suture placement. However, microanastomoses performed in free flap head and neck reconstruction represent only a specialized field. Other kinds of microsurgical procedures are commonly performed by the otolaryngologist, such as laryngeal and otologic surgeries. The four exercises were indeed chosen to allow the assessment of elementary microsurgery skills that are applicable to a vast majority of ENT surgical procedures.

Twenty-two medical students were included in the first phase.[9] The students were randomized into two different groups based on the different VITOM holding systems. In particular, 14 students performed the simulation using the

VERSACRANE (Karl Storz, Tuttlingen, Germany) holding system, while eight students used the ARTip cruise robotic holding arm (Karl Storz, Tuttlingen, Germany). All students successfully completed the training, and no technical issues were raised during the simulation. One student did not complete the microlaryngeal test due to the loss of the cottonoid during the task. We demonstrated that exoscope-based simulation is absolutely feasible and a good option for future training programs. The exoscope represents a slighter and more easily portable visualization system if compared to a surgical microscope, with potential advantages for training session organization. Further economic analysis should be performed to compare these tools in a training setting other than in the clinical context. Given the lower cost of the exoscope compared to the more sophisticated microscopes, training programs could benefit from this technology during course organization. Microsurgical courses are usually conducted with older microscopes to reduce the overall costs, and the lower quality of the visualization could have a potential impact on the training in a few days course. The exoscope could represent the right compromise in this context. Additional considerations should be done for the ARTip cruise robotic arm. No clear differences were highlighted between the two holding arms in performing the exercises. The better precision that could be obtained using a motorized arm is accompanied by a greater slowness of the movements. However, there are no differences in terms of visualization and magnification for obvious reasons. Moreover, the ARTip cruise system is a more cumbersome holding arm, similarly to the operating microscope. Finally, the VERSACRANE holding system is cheaper, and it surely represents the best compromise for microsurgery training at this time.

2.2.2 Preclinical comparison between the 3D exoscope and the operating microscope

Twenty eight consecutive medical students were included in the second phase of the study. The same four exercises were performed using the VITOM 3D exoscope mounted on the VERSACRANE holding system (Karl Storz, Tuttlingen, Germany) and the operating microscope (Zeiss OPMI CS NC31). All students were randomized in a cross-over design. A postintervention cross-sectional survey was also conducted to assess the overall quality of the simulation. The main features of a surgical visualization and magnification technology were assessed using a tailored questionnaire. We demonstrated that first-time users prefer the exoscope rather the operating microscope, particularly for "focusing" and "image quality." Moreover, the exoscope allows first-time users to better perform basic microsurgical tasks in a simulated clinical scenario when compared to the operating microscope. In particular, the time needed to perform each task using the two tools was compared. Although no significant difference was found in two exercises (*microlaryngeal test* and *gauze test*), the *maneuvering test* and the *pterional model test* have been performed more easily with the exoscope. In particular, the main challenge of the *pterional model test* was to repeatedly change the focus during the exercise to obtain a good visualization of the metal bars located at different depths. The exoscope could be easily controlled using the IMAGE1 PILOT, and the students had a free hand able to maintain surgical instruments during the task. Finally, the overall quality of the simulation was judged "very good" by the majority of the students (92.6%), demonstrating the feasibility and the reliability of the training and the tasks.

2.3 Preclinical application in laryngeal surgery

All new technologies and surgical instruments need a preclinical assessment and validation to define their applicability and reliability in clinical practice. The exoscope could be used in a simulation setting to improve the ability of first-time users in performing basic microsurgical tasks, as explained earlier. However, further applications could be proposed also for experienced surgeons.

Surgeons with hundreds of microsurgical procedures performed with the microscope have no technical issues with the procedure per se. If the exoscope is used as the surgical visualization and magnification tool, no major differences are encountered in terms of surgical instruments or surgical steps. However, an adaptation process should be taken into account, and the possibility to reduce its clinical impact on the surgical outcome should not be underestimated.

We developed several clinical scenarios that could be associated with the most common surgical procedures in the otolaryngology daily practice. A preclinical study was performed involving students, residents, and ENT specialists to test the feasibility of microlaryngeal surgery using the VITOM 3D-ARTip cruise system. The same *microlaryngeal test* previously described in this chapter was performed by three medical students, four ENT residents, and three ENT specialists. All ENT specialists had previous experience of VITOM 3D assisted surgery. All residents and students observed at least 10 cases of exoscope-assisted microlaryngeal surgery in a real clinical scenario, but they never used it. On the other hand, none in the sample had previous experience of the ARTip cruise robotic system, which was still not on the market at the time of the preclinical study. Different from the previous study, the time needed to position the VITOM 3D using the ARTip cruise robotic system at a distance of about 40 cm from the glottic plane.

All procedures were completed successfully without any delays or complaints. Although a direct comparison between groups was not possible due to the small sample, we observed that students and residents collected higher positioning times when compared with the ENT staff members. The ENT staff had previous experience with the IMAGE 1 pilot joystick that is used for the VITOM 3D optic settings in our routine practice and were surely facilitated in the ARTip cruise robotic system control. This also means that the potential gap between groups could be bridged after appropriate training. On the other hand, no great differences in terms of procedure times were collected between students, residents, and ENT staff. Finally, a tailored questionnaire was filled out by all participants after the procedure. The high movement precision, the ergonomics, and the improved visualization for all the OR members were judged as the main advantages of the VITOM 3D-ARTip cruise system.

2.4 Exoscope-based training in the OR

Exoscopic technology allows for an immersive education for fellows, residents, and students.[10] The key point to the educational benefits is that other members of the operating room can have the same view of the surgical site of the main operator. This was previously impossible with older operating microscopes. Although newer microscopes offer a second screen so that other operating room members can observe the surgical procedure, it is probably inferior in its teaching opportunities if compared to the exoscope. In particular, the image quality provided by the screen coupled with the microscope is surely inferior in terms of definition and contrast if compared to the main surgeon's view.

On the other hand, the exoscope provides the same quality of vision to surgeons, assistants, and students, giving the possibility to enjoy a visual perception of the surgical field, anatomic details, and microsurgical technique in a more realistic and surgeon-oriented way. Another factor that improves the educational role of the exoscope is that the main surgeon should not stay positioned at the eyepieces of a microscope. Therefore, he is able to freely gesture and explain to the other OR members the procedure, switching his gaze to the surgical sight with ease. Finally, the senior surgeon could easily guide the residents and fellows during the surgical procedure, following their movement with ease while looking at the same screen.

Some limitations should be pointed out from this perspective. The optimal 3D vision could be achieved only with the gaze perpendicular to the screen. Therefore, all the observers in the operating room should be positioned behind the main surgeon to benefit from its real view (Fig. 2.3A). Unfortunately, this would limit the number of students/residents that could observe the procedure simultaneously. However, additional screens with the same image quality could be placed in other positions in the OR to overcome this issue (Fig. 2.3B).

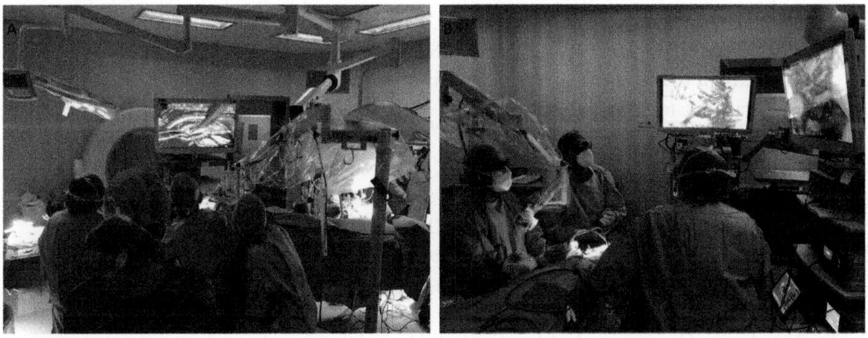

FIGURE 2.3

Operating room setting during exoscope-assisted microvascular anastomosis (A) and ear surgery (B).

2.5 Pearls and pitfalls

- The exoscope is a reliable tool for first time users in the microsurgery training setting.
- The exoscope allows first-time users to better perform basic microsurgical tasks in a simulated clinical scenario when compared to the operating microscope.
- First-time users prefer the exoscope rather than the operating microscope, particularly for "focusing" and "image quality."
- The high movement precision and the ergonomics are the main advantages of the VITOM 3D-ARTip *cruise* system in microlaryngeal surgery.
- Exoscopic technology provides the same quality of vision to all operating room members, giving the possibility to enjoy a visual perception of the surgical field, anatomic details, and microsurgical technique in a more realistic and surgeon-oriented way.
- The optimal 3D vision could be achieved only with the gaze perpendicular to the screen, and additional screens may be placed in other positions in the operating room to overcome this issue.
- The advent of exoscope-based microsurgical training with surely expedite the widespread of this new technology in the near future.

References

1. Tamai S. History of microsurgery. *Plast Reconstr Surg*. 2009;124(6 Suppl):e282–294.
2. Evgeniou E, Walker H, Gujral S. The role of simulation in microsurgical training. *J Surg Educ*. 2018;75(1):171–181.
3. Gardner AK, Scott DJ, Hebert JC, et al. Gearing up for milestones in surgery: will simulation play a role? *Surgery*. 2015;158(5):1421–1427.
4. Javid P, Aydın A, Mohanna P-N, Dasgupta P, Ahmed K. Current status of simulation and training models in microsurgery: a systematic review. *Microsurgery*. 2019;39(7):655–668.
5. De Virgilio A, Mercante G, Gaino F, et al. Preliminary clinical experience with the 4 K3-dimensional microvideoscope (VITOM 3D) system for free flap head and neck reconstruction. *Head Neck*. 2020;42(1):138–140.
6. Smith S, Kozin ED, Kanumuri VV, et al. Initial experience with 3-dimensional exoscope-assisted transmastoid and lateral skull base surgery. *Otolaryngol Head Neck Surg*. 2019;160(2):364–367.
7. Ricciardi L, Chaichana KL, Cardia A, et al. The exoscope in neurosurgery: an innovative "point of view". A systematic review of the technical, surgical and educational aspects. *World Neurosurg*. 2019. S1878-8750(19)30080-30084.
8. De Virgilio A, Costantino A, Mondello T, et al. Pre-clinical experience with the VITOM 3D and the ARTip cruise system for micro-laryngeal surgery. *Laryngoscope*. 2021;131(1):136–138.
9. De Virgilio A, Costantino A, Ebm C, et al. High definition three-dimensional exoscope (VITOM 3D) for microsurgery training: a preliminary experience. *Eur Arch Otorhinolaryngol*. 2020;277(9):2589–2595.
10. Ricciardi L, Mattogno PP, Olivi A, Sturiale CL. Exoscope era: next technical and educational step in microneurosurgery. *World Neurosurg*. 2019;128:371–373.

CHAPTER

Exoscope-assisted microlaryngeal surgery

3

Armando De Virgilio, MD, PhD [1], Elena Russo, MD [2,3], Andrea Costantino, MD [2,3], Giovanni Cugini, MD [3], Giuseppe Spriano, MD [4]

[1]*Assistant Professor of Otorhinolaryngology-Head and Neck Surgery, Humanitas University, Milan, Italy;* [2]*Department of Biomedical Sciences, Humanitas University, Pieve Emanuele, Milan, Italy;* [3]*Otorhinolaryngology Unit, IRCCS Humanitas Clinical and Research Center, Rozzano, Milan, Italy;* [4]*Professor and Chief of Otorhinolaryngology-Head and Neck Surgery, Humanitas University, Milan, Italy*

3.1 The introduction of exoscopes in microlaryngeal surgery

The use of the operating microscope in laryngology was first introduced in 1960 by Scalco, Shipman, and Tabb in New Orleans, United States.[1] In their work, they described the applicability of a Zeiss binocular microscope, designed for otologic surgery, with the Lynch suspension laryngoscope to treat small, benign lesions, confined to the true vocal folds. However, it is up to Oskar Kleinsasser to have refined the methodic and to have spread it from 1968 onwards throughout the world.[2] Indeed, the technique, as described by Scalco and colleagues, showed several limits: the magnification was inadequate, the equipment was unwieldy, and the customary laryngoscopes were not suitable for binocular vision. Furthermore, the short focal length of the Zeiss microscope was not adequate for long-shafted laryngeal instruments. In this scenario, Dr. Kleinsasser has developed a laryngoscope larger and tapered, thus allowing to accomplish the binocular vision and bimanual surgery.[3,4] By the same time, Zeiss had introduced a 400 mm focal lens that permitted an easier use of the long steeled laryngeal instruments for precision surgery of the vocal folds with vastly improved functional results.

Microlaryngeal surgery nowadays (MLS) is a technique that provides for direct examination of the larynx as well as for treatment of benign and malign diseases of the larynx and phonomicrosurgery, using an operating microscope. The use of an operating microscope is preferred over an external surgical approach as it is far less invasive and leads to significantly less intraoperative and postoperative complications such as damage to the blood vessels with consequent significant blood loss, damage to the nerves (particularly CN X) leading to dysphonia and dysphagia, scarring, and postoperative wound infections. MLS also reduces the operating time, the length of hospitalization, and the length of recovery for the patient, thus also bringing economic benefits to the hospital and health benefits to the patient.

Exoscope-Assisted Surgery in Otorhinolaryngology. https://doi.org/10.1016/B978-0-323-83168-0.00011-2

MLS is performed under general anesthesia. The operating laryngoscope (Kleinsasser laryngoscope) is used to expose the vocal folds. The patient is laid in a supine position with the head slightly hyperextended, and the operating microscope is positioned behind the patient's head. The laryngoscope is attached to a laryngosuspension apparatus consisting of an adjustable rod anchored to the operating bed. Microlaryngoscopy can be performed with either "cold" instruments or with a CO_2 laser.

Although the traditional operating microscope is an essential surgical instrument to perform fine and delicate surgeries, like microlaryngeal surgery, technological advancements have introduced the exoscope as a potential substitute.[5–8] Karl Storz's video telescope operating monitor or "VITOM" was released in 2011. Originally, it was equipped only with 2D platforms, while the VITOM 3D exoscope was launched in 2017.

In 2012, Carlucci et al. first described the use of an exoscope in endoscopic laryngeal surgery.[9] They treated 12 patients with benign and malign pathologies of the vocal folds, using a telescope (VITOM, Karl Storz) equipped with a high-definition endoscopic video system, showing its potential advantages in terms of ease and comfort of the surgeon.

This chapter aims to describe thoroughly the technical characteristics of the exoscopic microlaryngeal surgery, analyzing its feasibility and suitability, with a particular mention to the authors' experience.

3.2 Surgical procedure and setting

The patient is in a supine position with the head extended on the neck and the neck flexed on the chest (Boyce–Jackson position). General anesthesia is carried out through orotracheal intubation and the operating laryngoscope is used to expose the glottic plane, and then attached to a fulcrum-type laryngosuspension apparatus, consisting of an adjustable rod anchored to the operating table. The VITOM 3D operating exoscope mounted on the VERSACRANE holding system is placed behind the patient's head, about 35–45 cm from the operating field (Fig. 3.1).

The vertical column equipped with the monitor (IMAGE1 S platform) and the light source is placed in front of the main surgeon, sitting behind the patient's head, while the scrub nurse stands on the right side of the patient. The assistant surgeon can position himself or herself on the left side of the patient's head. From this position, he or she is able to constantly adjust the framing and the focusing of the image, thanks to the IMAGE1 PILOT control joystick, by looking at the same 3D-HD screen. At the same time, the assistant surgeon can hold the suction or other surgical instruments and can make external counterpressure on the larynx, if needed. Indeed, when it is not possible to visualize the vocal folds up to the anterior commissure, it is possible to optimize such exposure using different maneuvers, such as external laryngeal counterpressure and flexion–flexion position. Other operating room (OR) members, such as students, should position themselves behind the main surgeon to maintain a perpendicular view of the screen. The disposition of

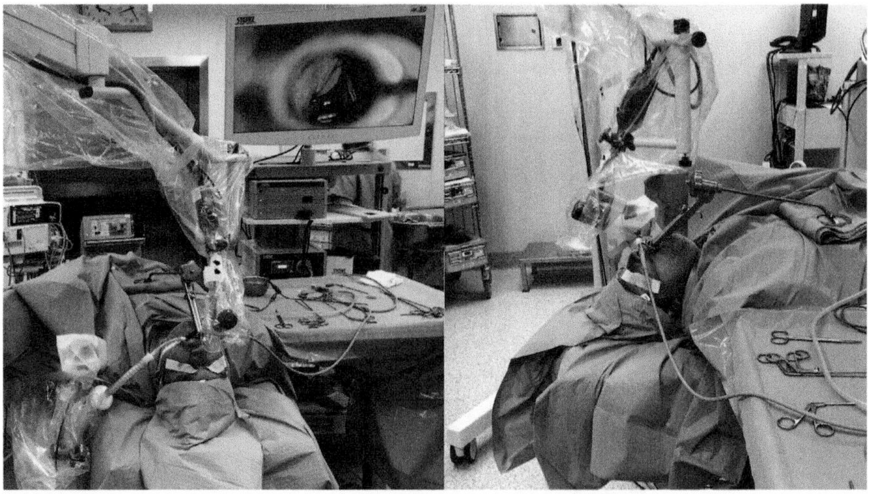

FIGURE 3.1

Frontal and lateral view of VITOM 3D setting in microlaryngeal surgery.

the nurse's master table and secondary table, as well as the anesthesia device or other surgical devices in the OR, is not further influenced by the application of this setting and is totally similar to a traditional procedure.

The basic setup of the operating room is shown in Fig. 3.2.

3.2.1 Surgical instruments

The surgical instruments that can be used under exoscopic control are the same as those used with the operating microscope. The classical phonosurgical set including a variety of forceps and scissors specifically designed for MLS, as well as a long and small caliber aspirator to provide suction of blood, sputum, and debris can be used. As previously mentioned, MLS can be performed with either "cold" instruments or with a CO_2 laser, which is crucial as a cutting device, in transoral laser microsurgery for laryngeal tumors. Recently, Carobbio et al. first described the application of a coupling system (model TH004 Micromanipulator Interface VITOM; Karl Storz SE & Co. KG, Tuttlingen, Germany) allowing the use of VITOM 3D-HD viewing platform together with the free-beam laser CO_2 laser micromanipulator, which is usually fixed to the microscope.[10] This system replaces the microscope head with a new adaptor piece that positions the VITOM 3D-HD horizontally, providing for a free line of sight in front of the surgeon. Chapter 4 describes in detail CO_2 laser endoscopic-assisted laryngeal surgery.

3.2.2 Indications

The pathological conditions that can be treated with this technique are the same as traditional MLS: papillomatosis, cysts, nodules, polyps, Reinke's edema, granuloma,

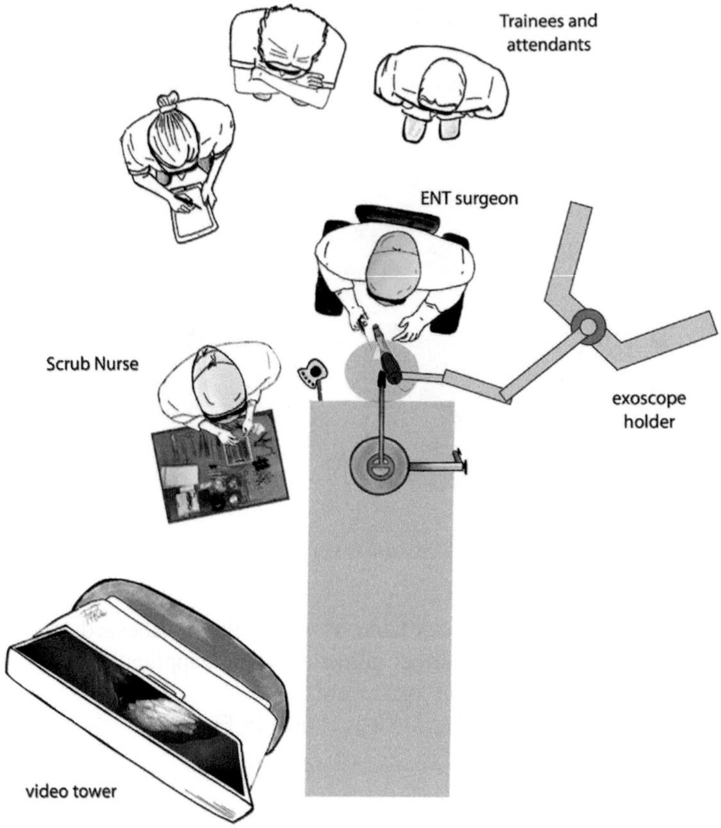

FIGURE 3.2

Operating room setup in microlaryngeal surgery.

leukoplakia, dysplasia, cancer, scar, sulcus and vergeture, vascular lesion, glottic web, and vocal fold paralysis (augmentation).

3.3 Our experience

Between April 2019 and May 2020, a total of 45 consecutive patients (males: 29; median age: 57.0 years, IQR 43.0–65.0) diagnosed with laryngeal lesions treatable without laser were enrolled at our institution (Humanitas Clinical and Research Center, Rozzano, MI). The VITOM 3D exoscope mounted on the VERSACRANE holding system (Karl Storz, Tuttlingen, Germany) was used to perform all the procedures.

Thirteen (28.8%) patients presented a malignant lesion. The most frequent benign pathology was vocal cord polyps ($n = 16$, 35.5%). The remaining patients

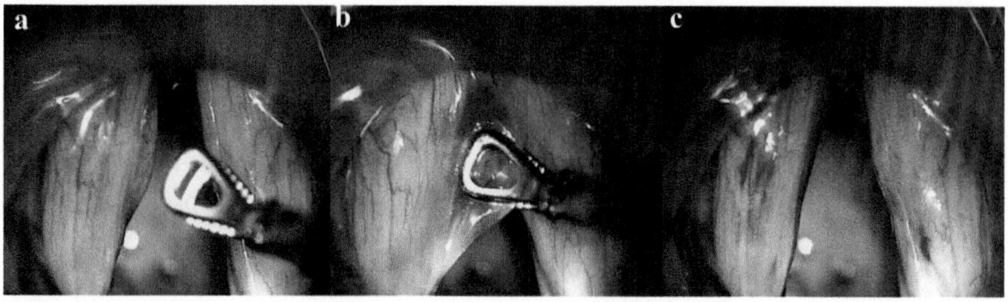

FIGURE 3.3

Vocal polyp excision using the VITOM 3D: (A) polyp magnification; (B) polyp traction using the bouchayer-type forceps; (C) complete excision.

suffered from vocal cord cyst ($n = 5$, 11.1%), Reinke's edema ($n = 3$, 6.6%), vocal cord lesion ($n = 2$, 4.4%), vocal cord nodules ($n = 2$, 4.4%), vocal cord leukoplakia ($n = 2$, 4.4%), laryngeal granuloma ($n = 1$, 2.2%), and laryngeal papilloma ($n = 1$, 2.2%). As a consequence, the majority of the procedures were therapeutic ($n = 32$, 71.1%, e.g., Fig. 3.3), while the remaining were diagnostic ($n = 13$, 28.9%).

All surgeries were successfully completed without the need for the operating microscope, and no complications or unwanted delays were expressed by the surgeons or scrub nurses. An adequate view of the surgical field was achieved through the VITOM, and it did not pose any obstacle to surgery. The VITOM successfully produced a high-resolution stereoscopic image of the surgical field with the use of polarized 3D glasses. All surgical instruments traditionally used in MLS with an operating microscope were used with the exoscope, without any issues.

3.4 Advantages and disadvantages

Our case series demonstrate the feasibility of microlaryngeal surgery using the VITOM 3D exoscope. All surgeries were successfully completed without the support of the operating microscope, and no complications or unwanted delays were expressed neither by the surgeons or the scrub nurses.

To better understand the differences between the operating microscope and the exoscope, we investigated the advantages and disadvantages of the VITOM 3D exoscope in this specific clinical setting.

Compared with the conventional operating microscope, the VITOM 3D exoscope mounted on the VERSACRANE holding system is smaller and does not encumber the operating field. This allows the surgeon to perform microlaryngeal surgery in a more natural posture, thus reducing his or her fatigue and physical discomfort during the procedure. Visualization of the surgical field is not limited to the eyepieces, as the image is projected onto a large monitor, thus allowing for a neutral cervical spine posture. Indeed, one of the major complaints when working with the operating microscope is the need to remain in a fixed position to see through the lens. In addition, this view is often disrupted as the operator frequently has to look away to change surgical instruments and to give instructions to other members of the surgical staff, as well as to readjust the focus. The VITOM has a greater depth of field than the operating microscope. One study reported the VITOM's depth of field as 3.5–10 cm compared to the operating microscope's <1.2 cm.[11] This explains why the operators who performed using the operating microscope have to more frequently focus the lenses when compared to those who used the VITOM.

The holding system allows for a focal distance from 20 to 50 cm, depending on the surgical procedure. The VITOM's camera is very small and can be positioned high above the surgical site, thanks to its high focal length (Fig. 3.4).

In exoscopic microlaryngeal surgery, the optimal distance of the exoscope from the operating field is between 35 and 45 cm. This provides a sufficiently wide working space, thus allowing the surgeon to operate with more free and easy motions, and to use a classical set of phonosurgical microinstruments, such as triangular Bouchayer forceps, curved alligators, microscissors, microaspirators, and endoscopic needles for intracordal injections.

Difficult laryngeal exposure may limit the utility of MLS in certain patients. The VERSACRANE holding system had greater maneuverability than most of the operating microscopes: many joints of this system can be manually adjusted by the operator to place the camera in many different positions, allowing for visualization of complex viewing angles. Moreover, the precision of the 3D camera can be further improved using the ARTip *cruise* robotic system.[12] This motorized holding arm provides a more stable view of the operating field and allows the operator to reach difficult viewing angles, thanks to a pivot movement around the focal point.

Unlike the operating microscope, the exoscope's 3D camera does not have an adjustable telescopic lens, thus resulting in a loss of image quality. Indeed, the

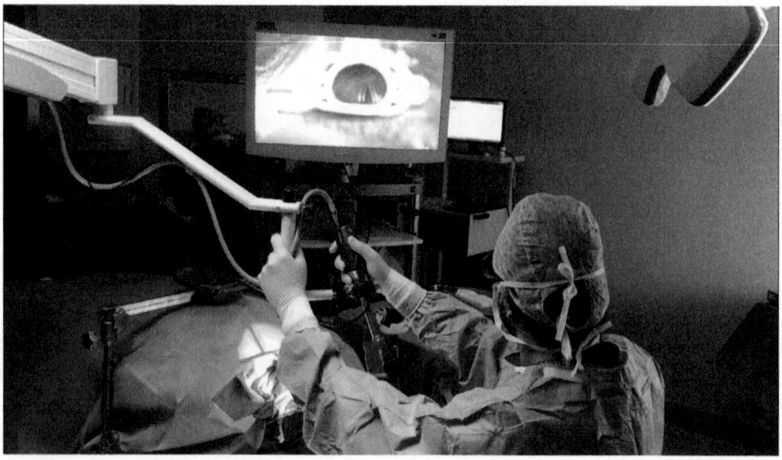

FIGURE 3.4

VITOM 3D placement using the VERSACRANE holding system.

surgical image is gradually blurred as the magnification rate increases. Nevertheless, MLS does not usually require the maximum magnification power of 30×. Moreover, the new exoscopic systems project images at 4K resolution, thus making negligible the loss of resolution during magnification.

Many surgeons use the microscope to obtain a stereoscopic view. As aforementioned, the first models of VITOM worked with only one camera and therefore the image was only in 2D. This led to many surgeons complaining about a loss of depth perception.[13] This was a major change in the VITOM 3D models as it operates with two cameras, thus providing visualization of the surgical field in three dimensions.

Illumination of the surgical field is extremely important. Low light levels can obscure the image and lead to much difficulty while operating. It is particularly important for operating with a small surgical field and where the color chromaticity can be lost by poor lighting. The light source is built into the VITOM, being about 1.5 cm from the camera, and it comes from the tabletop light source. It is worth noting that this distance from the light to the camera can lead to an inaccurate positioning of the light, especially when a small-sized Kleinsasser laryngoscope is used or when the camera is positioned near to the surgical field. Furthermore, the VITOM's rays of light are quite widely spread and not focused on a point, thus affecting the surgical field luminance. The use of a Xenon light in the place of an LED light may increase the luminance. However, the drawback of the Xenon light is that it increases the temperature of the surgical field a lot more than the lamps, leading to potential thermal injury of the involved tissue.[14]

3.5 Conclusions

The exoscope could be used as a safe and valuable alternative to the operating microscope in microlaryngeal surgery. The ergonomics is probably the main advantage of this system, together with the ease of using and the educational potential, due to the possibility to share the same surgical image among all the OR members. On the other hand, the image quality, and particularly the luminance of the surgical field, could represent a limit for MLS, especially in first-time users. As a consequence, further technological advancements are required to improve some technical characteristics of this system, such as the quality of the image and its brightness. Finally, the recent introduction of a system to couple the VITOM 3D-HD with the free-beam CO_2 laser micromanipulator will surely make this technology even more widespread and appreciated.

- The exoscope could be safely used in MLS, representing a valuable alternative to the surgical microscope.
- The operating room setup is fairly different compared to traditional microscope-based MLS, while the patient's position and surgical instruments are the same.
- The exoscope is adequate to treat all pathological conditions commonly treated with microscope-based MLS.

- The ergonomics, the ease of using, and the educational potential are the main advantages of this system.
- The image quality and the luminance of the surgical field may require further technical improvements.

References

1. Scalco AN, Shipman WF, Tabb HG. Microscopic suspension laryngoscopy. *Ann Otol Rhinol Laryngol*. 1960;69:1134–1138.
2. Menon UK. A historical review of laryngology. In: *Textbook of Laryngology*. 1st ed. New Delhi: Jaypee Brothers Medical Publishers; 2017.
3. Kleinsasser O. [A laryngomicroscope for the early diagnosis and differential diagnosis of cancers in the larynx, pharynx and mouth]. *Z Laryngol Rhinol Otol*. 1961;40:276–279.
4. Kleinsasser O. Mikrolaryngoskopie und endolaryngeale Mikrochirurgie. I. Technische Entwicklung der Methode [Microlaryngoscopy and endolaryngeal microsurgery. I. Technical development of the method (author's transl)]. *HNO*. 1974;22(2):33–38.
5. Mamelak AN, Danielpour M, Black KL, Hagike M, Berci G. A high-definition exoscope system for neurosurgery and other microsurgical disciplines: preliminary report. *Surg Innov*. 2008;15(1):38–46.
6. Ricciardi L, Chaichana KL, Cardia A, et al. The exoscope in neurosurgery: an innovative "point of view". A systematic review of the technical, surgical and educational aspects. *World Neurosurg*. 2019. S1878-8750(19)30080-30084.
7. Ichikawa Y, Senda D, Shingyochi Y, Mizuno H. Potential advantages of using three-dimensional exoscope for microvascular anastomosis in free flap transfer. *Plast Reconstr Surg*. 2019;144(4):726e–727e.
8. Piatkowski AA, Keuter XHA, Schols RM, van der Hulst RRWJ. Potential of performing a microvascular free flap reconstruction using solely a 3D exoscope instead of a conventional microscope. *J Plast Reconstr Aesthet Surg*. 2018;71(11):1664–1678.
9. Carlucci C, Fasanella L, Ricci Maccarini A. Exolaryngoscopy: a new technique for laryngeal surgery. *Acta Otorhinolaryngol Ital*. 2012;32(5):326–328.
10. Carobbio ALC, Filauro M, Parrinello G, Missale F, Peretti G. Microsurgical procedures during COVID-19 pandemic: the VITOM® 3D-HD exoscopic system as alternative to the operating microscope to properly use personal protective equipment (PPE). *Eur Arch Otorhinolaryngol*. 2020. https://doi.org/10.1007/s00405-020-06239-6.
11. Oertel JM, Burkhardt BW. Vitom-3D for exoscopic neurosurgery: initial experience in cranial and spinal procedures. *World Neurosurg*. 2017;105:153–162.
12. De Virgilio A, Costantino A, Mondello T, et al. Pre-clinical experience with the VITOM 3D and the ARTip cruise system for micro-laryngeal surgery. *Laryngoscope*. 2021; 131(1):136–138.
13. Nishiyama K. From exoscope into the next generation. *J Korean Neurosurg Soc*. 2017; 60(3):289–293.
14. Sato T, Bakhit MS, Suzuki K, et al. Utility and safety of a novel surgical microscope laser light source. *PLoS One*. 2018;13(2):e0192112.

CHAPTER

Exoscope-assisted laser laryngeal surgery

4

Giorgio Peretti, MD [1,2], Andrea Luigi Camillo Carobbio, MD [1,2,3], Giampiero Parrinello, MD [1], Francesco Missale, MD [1,4]

[1]*IRCCS Ospedale Policlinico San Martino, Genova, Italy;* [2]*Department of Surgical Sciences and Integrated Diagnostics (DISC), University of Genoa, Genoa, Italy;* [3]*Section of Otorhinolaryngology, Head and Neck Surgery – Azienda Ospedaliera di Padova, University of Padua, Padua, Italy;* [4]*Department of Molecular and Translational Medicine, University of Brescia, Brescia, Italy*

4.1 The exoscope in transoral laryngeal surgery

4.1.1 Background

The recent development of exoscopic systems was first aimed for surgical recording and teaching purposes. Then, the implementation with 3D cameras, 4K resolution, and ergonomic holders have driven increasing interest in their application for direct surgical view. In the head and neck field, several applications have been tested, including otosurgery, otoneurosurgery, microvascular anastomosis, and transoral oropharyngeal surgery.[1–5] These studies have demonstrated the easy use of the exoscopic camera as a magnifier, without any coupling system for the correct use of a cutting device paired with the viewing system. In all clinical scenarios tested, the exoscopic camera presents the advantage of video recording for teaching purposes and the possibility for the entire surgical team to get the same 3D view of the main surgeon. Moreover, the surgeon's ergonomics was improved compared to conventional microsurgery.

The idea of replacing the operating microscope during transoral laryngeal microsurgery,[6,7] introduced the issue of how to combine a CO_2 laser micromanipulator, not yet available for the previously proposed exoscopic systems. For this reason, in collaboration with the engineers of the Italian Technology Institute (IIT) we developed a coupler device suitable for the use of the free-beam CO_2 laser micromanipulator combined with a 3D-HD exoscopic system.[8,9]

Exoscope-Assisted Surgery in Otorhinolaryngology. https://doi.org/10.1016/B978-0-323-83168-0.00005-7

4.2 Our experience: the road toward a feasible exoscope-TLM setting

4.2.1 First prototype holder arm with VITOM 3D

4.2.1.1 Surgical setting

The idea of overcoming the limitations of the operative microscope and fully replicate a transoral laser microsurgery (TOLMS) setting, coupling the free-beam CO_2 laser micromanipulator with the new exoscopic system, radically changed the system of visualization and led to novel difficulties and shortcomings. In fact, the technologies employed were not conceived to be assembled in a transoral microsurgical setting. To make them work efficiently as a whole, several adaptations were needed, especially in terms of stability, paring, and movement.

As an exoscopic system of vision, the VITOM 3D-HD (Karl Storz SE & Co. KG, Tuttlingen, Germany) was employed.[8] Since it was conceived to enhance visualization quality in micro and open surgical procedures, the VITOM 3D-HD was equipped with a thin and lightweight holding system called VERSACRANE LIGHT. While being very compact and wieldy to hold the VITOM in position, the VERSACRANE did not have sufficient stability when the first tests with the laser micromanipulator were carried out. In particular, many vibrations affecting the frame resulted in unstable vision during laser positioning and movements, probably due to the extra weight of the manipulator that the holding system was not designed to support. This issue revealed the necessity to substitute the VERSACRANE with a new holder, specifically conceived to firmly support the weight of the VITOM and micromanipulator simultaneously in a transoral laser microsurgical setting. Thus, a customized support arm (Fig. 4.1) was created in collaboration with the IIT, designed to be

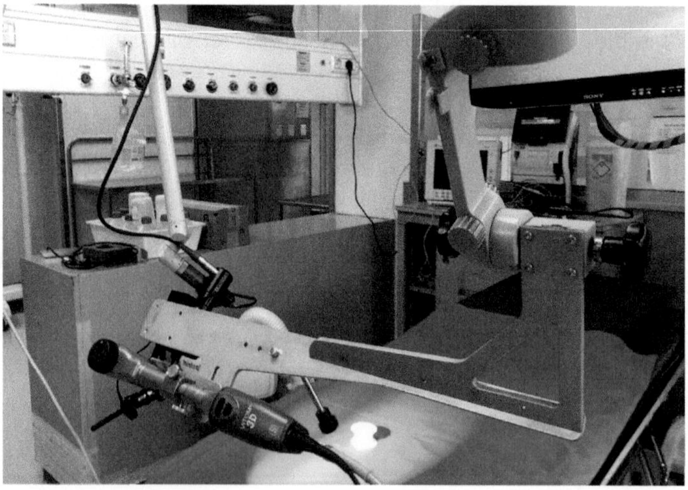

FIGURE 4.1

The customized support arm holding the VITOM 3D-HD.

mounted on a Zeiss microscope stative, removing the optic system. The holder arm was provided with a handle to allow macroscopic movements and positioning, knobs to lock all joints in place once the definitive position of the support structure was reached, and a specific regulatory wheel for precise adjustments of the framing angle. A specific adaptor plate (model TH004 Micromanipulator Interface VITOM, installation of CO_2 laser micromanipulators on VITOM 3; Karl Storz SE & Co. KG, Tuttlingen, Germany) was designed by IIT engineers and fixed to the holder arm to allow for coupling with the micromanipulator, so that the micromanipulator could be stably fixed in a position aligned with the line of sight of the VITOM 3D-HD.

With this prototype of the exoscope-assisted transoral laser microsurgical setting, the essential requisites for precise alignment between the line of sight of the exoscope through the laryngoscope and laser micromanipulator workspace were achieved. Moreover, the ideal operating distance between the laser scanner and surgical target was precisely established to optimize the "char-free" cutting properties of the laser. The methods followed for these adjustments are thoroughly described in a previous publication.[8]

Besides helping the first surgeon in traditional TOLM with external counterpressure on the larynx and cooperating to a surgical maneuver with suction or other surgical tools, with the exoscopic system the assistant surgeon can constantly follow the procedure on the 3D surgical screen and, if needed, zoom in on a particular target, regulate focus, and slightly move the framing to follow the first surgeon's maneuvers using the IMAGE1 PILOT control device, directly fixed on the left side of the operating bed (see also Chapter 1).

The preliminary results with this novel prototype in alternative to the traditional TOLMS, were obtained in 17 nonconsecutive oncological cases.[8]

4.2.1.2 Adaptability to fiber laser procedures

An additional advantage of this setting can be employed by removing the CO2 laser micromanipulator from its adaptor plate on the VITOM holder arm and using a fiber laser with different wavelength with less precise and char-free cut, but a better control of hemostasis, in relation to the site and type of resection. This offers the simultaneous availability to employ 3D angled telescopes for different indications or different surgical steps of the same procedure.

In our experience, a flexible fiber tulium/diode laser was utilized when the disease involved one of the supraglottic subsites in the presence of extensions to the medial hypopharyngeal wall or to the base of the tongue. During the preparation of this setting, a good suggestion is to move the exoscope slightly away from the laryngoscope/mouth-gag compared to the CO_2 laser setup, thereby offering a wider operative field and avoiding competition between surgical instruments, which is not easily feasible with the standard operative microscope.

4.2.1.3 Issues

Although being comparable to the traditional microscope setting once a good position and framing have been obtained, the currently described prototype setting for

CO_2 laser exoscope-assisted transoral procedures was still affected by some stability and movement fluency issues during manual positioning of the holder arm and macroscopic adjustments of the framing. Moreover, the full-HD vision technology employed had been already overcome by other devices equipped with 4K resolution and slightly higher image quality.

4.2.2 Adaptation for the ORBEYE system

4.2.2.1 From full-HD to 4K resolution

The same concept of an exoscope-assisted transoral surgical setting for the larynx was replicated with state-of-the-art technology in terms of vision, the ORBEYE 4K 3D platform (Sony Olympus Medical Solutions, Tokyo, Japan; FDA approved). This exoscope is characterized by one of the highest magnification powers (26× with the 55-in. screen), while maintaining full-size 4K image resolution along the entire range of available enlargements. Furthermore, it is equipped with a motorized support arm that makes its movements fluid, easy to maneuver, and accurate during the framing. The movements of the motorized arm can be controlled manually with simultaneous pressure on three buttons placed at the head of the arm and dragging it into position before the procedure starts. In addition, fine adjustments of the inclination, zoom, and focus of the image can be regulated by a pedal control with other adjunctive commands and customizable shortcuts.

Furthermore, the inclusion of the narrow band imaging (NBI) tool, developed in the gastroenterological setting and now widely used in the upper aerodigestive tract,[10] represents an adjunctive value allowing for real time intraoperative control of the superficial extension of the lesion and margins of resection. In the field of transoral laryngeal surgery, the high magnification power with 4K resolution and excellent lighting and image definition features permit a clear view even in the narrow corridor of a laryngoscope, ensuring precise phonomicrosurgical procedures with cold instruments or fiber laser resections, with better ergonomics.

4.2.2.2 Issues

The transoral setting with the ORBEYE system cannot be coupled with a CO_2 laser micromanipulator at this time, since this would require a specifically designed adaptor plate to be mounted on its motorized arm. For this reason, no transoral CO_2 laser procedure on the larynx can be performed with this setting, representing the most limiting factor to its application in exoscope-assisted transoral laser laryngeal surgery.

4.2.2.3 Adaptability to fiber laser procedures

Nonetheless, the ORBEYE system can fully replace the microscope when the surgeon chooses to use a fiber laser for the resection, particularly for the supraglottic larynx and/or hypopharynx. In this setting, the possibility for the surgeon to use both hands to manipulate laryngeal tissues and surgical instrumentation, while at the same time controlling the frame, zoom, focus, and additional features like NBI with his foot on the pedal represents a real step forward in terms of performance, ergonomics, and surgical experience.

4.2.2.4 *Case series*

Our experience is derived from a case series of 12 patients successfully treated in September 2019 with the ORBEYE exoscopic system. In particular, seven transoral procedures were performed with fiber laser (three tonsillectomies, three laryngeal tumors, one parapharyngeal tumor), three glottic phonomicrosurgical procedures with cold instrumentation, and two cases of free flap harvesting with microvascular anastomosis (Fig. 4.2).[11]

4.3 The VITOM-3D ARTip Cruise System

4.3.1 The intraoperative setting

To the best of our knowledge, among the current equipment able to perform exoscopic transoral free-beam laser-assisted microsurgery, the VITOM 3D-HD coupled with the electromechanic holder ARTip Cruise together with the support for a micromanipulator (model TH004 Micromanipulator Interface VITOM; Karl Storz SE & Co. KG, Tuttlingen, Germany), is the only exoscopic setting available on the market to apply this type surgery.

The abovementioned surgical setting is the end point of the research that resolved several limitations and weak points of previous solutions applied in preclinical research.

The system is composed of a full integration of a viewing system (VITOM 3D-HD) paired with a 32″ 3D monitor (model TM330, Karl Storz), a coupler device supporting and accurately pairing the VITOM 3D-HD with the free-beam CO_2 laser micromanipulator, and an ergonomic and motorized holder (ARTip Cruise) (Fig. 4.3).

The surgical procedure is carried out following the steps usually conducted during conventional transoral laser microsurgery (Fig. 4.4A). The diagnostic workup should include meticulous examination of the tumor, both during preoperative examination with flexible high definition videoendoscopes, and intraoperatively after laryngeal suspension with rigid scopes, both including biological endoscopy assessment. This meticulous diagnostic assessment is crucial to select patients who also require radiological evaluation (with CT or MRI), and to plan the resection ensuring the identification of safe superficial and deep margins. The use of diagnostic tools such as the Laryngoscore[12,13] is encouraged since it has previously been shown to accurately predict the probability of obtaining good intraoperative exposure that can guarantee the successful exploitation of the surgical procedure with a low rate of close and positive margins.[12] Its utility is further represented by the possibility of adequate preoperative counseling, avoiding intraoperative twists and granting the optimal choice of laryngoscopes.

After the conventional laryngeal suspension with direct eye view, the microscope is fully substituted by the VITOM-3D held by the ARTip Cruise System, which is placed on the right side of the first surgeon (Fig. 4.3A). The IMAGE1 PILOT used to control the zoom and the fine movements of the arm is placed on the left side, and it can also be reached by the assistant (Fig. 4.3A and C).

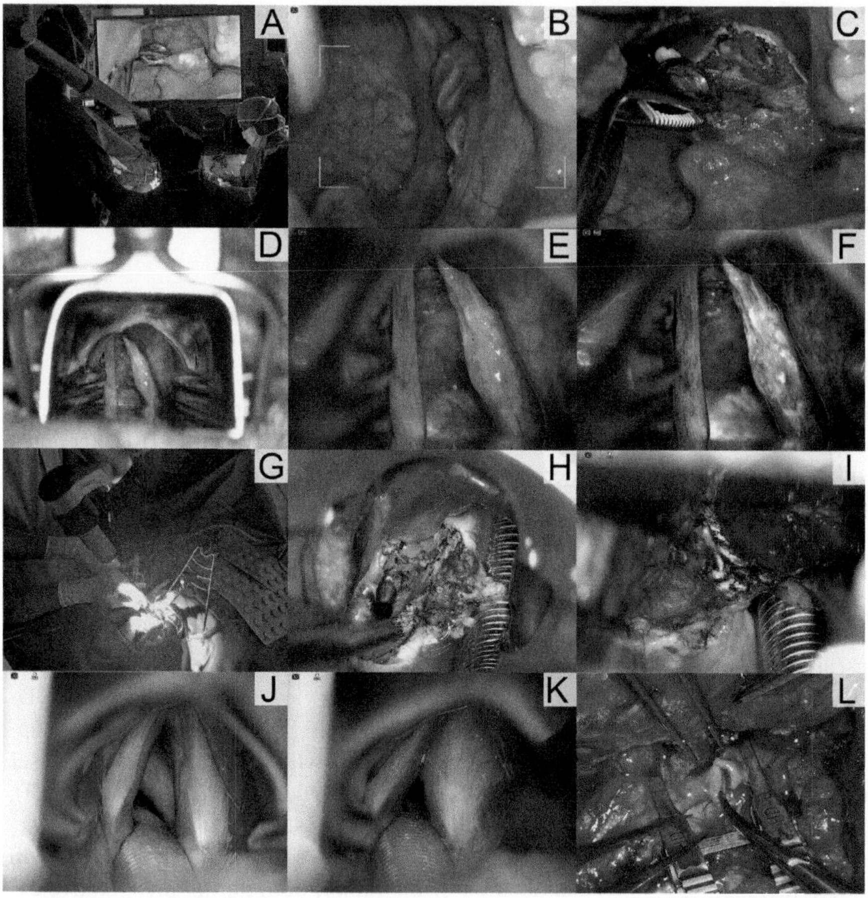

FIGURE 4.2

Representative applications of the ORBEYE 4K 3D. Surgical setting (A) and intraoperative view (B, C) of a transoral exoscopic tonsillectomy (A). Intraoperative view of a right vocal fold carcinoma seen through the narrow space of a laryngoscope with the ORBEYE 4K 3D exoscope (D); full magnification surgical view with white light (E), or enhanced with NBI (F). Surgical setting during a transoral exoscopic resection of a left benign parapharyngeal space tumor (G), the left pharyngotomy is necessary to approach the parapharyngeal space by fiber thulium-diode laser (H), and the dissection along the tumor capsule (I). Intraoperative view of the glottis before (J) and after (K) a right vocal fold augmentation with autologous fat. End-to-end microvascular anastomosis performed with the ORBEYE 4K 3D assistance during the insetting of a radial forearm free flap (L).

The camera can be first positioned by keeping the button on the arm pushed down, which releases its friction and moves it manually to obtain visualization of the surgical field. Given that the focal distance of the VITOM-3D is between 200

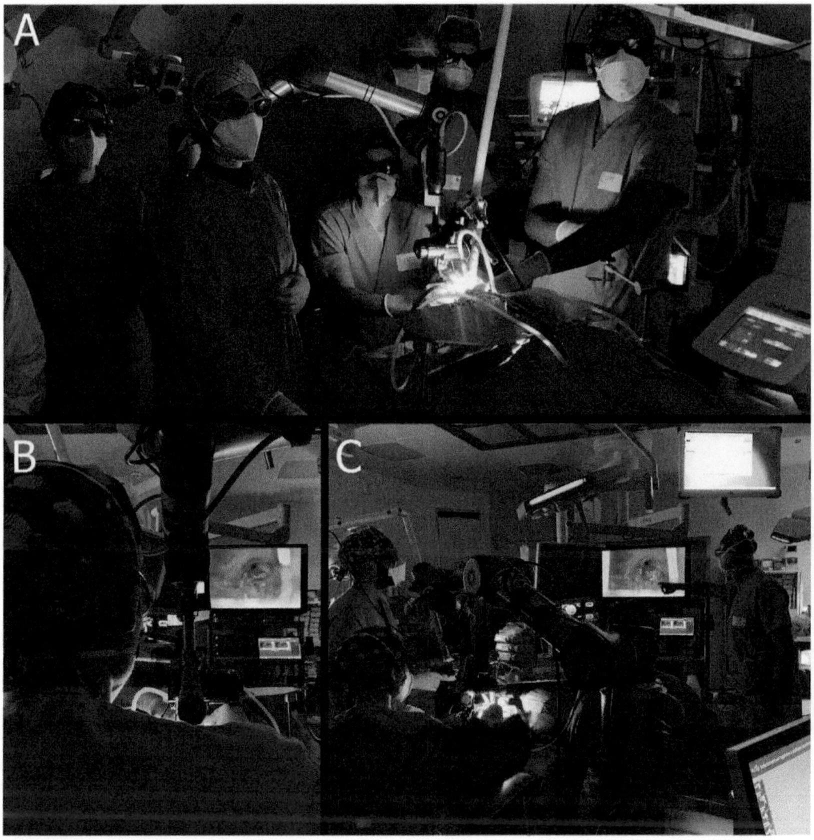

FIGURE 4.3

The VITOM 3D-HD ARTip Cruise free-beam CO_2 laser setting. Pictures of the surgical theater during an exoscopic CO_2 laser-assisted TOLM procedure. In (A), several observers can have the same 3D view of the first surgeon; (B) shows the view from the first surgeon position and in (C) the senior surgeon can guide the trainee giving suggestions pointing to the 32″ 3D monitor.

and 500 mm, and that the Digital AcuBlade working distances ranges between 250 and 400 mm, their coupled use is easily manageable, as previously described.[8] The main novelty of this setting compared with the previous experimental ones is the possibility to remotely and digitally control the fine movements of the mechanic arm with the IMAGE1 PILOT, managing both translation along the axial plane of view and rotations having the camera as fulcrum. Once the arm is roughly positioned centering the surgical field at low magnification, the desired magnification can be reached with the IMAGE1 PILOT, and fine movement control is obtained pushing

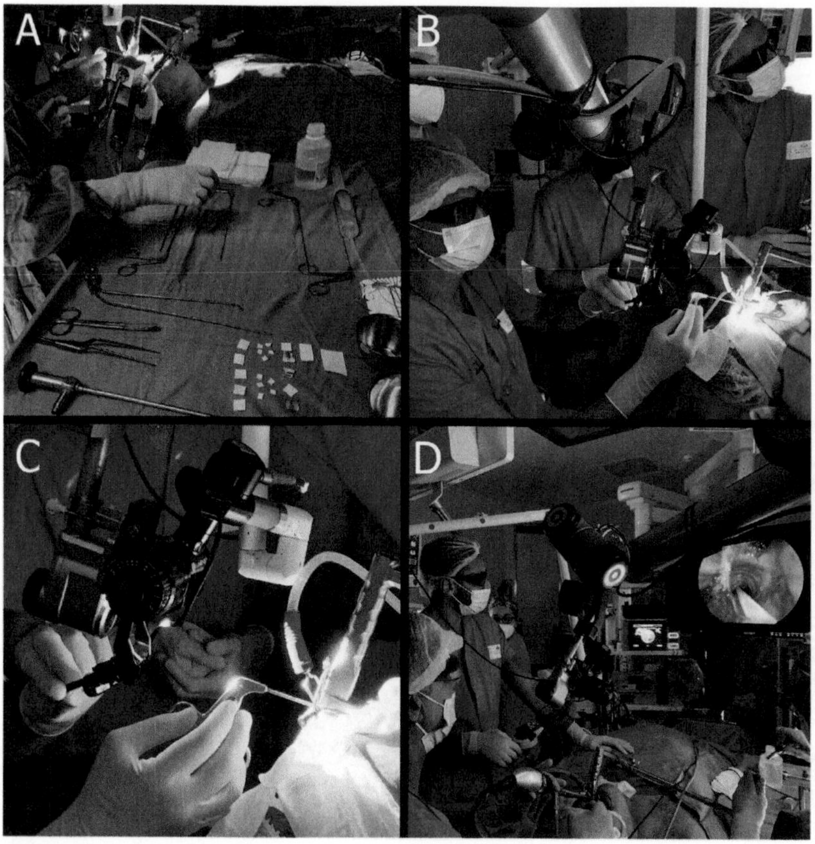

FIGURE 4.4

Details of the VITOM 3D-HD ARTip Cruise free-beam CO_2 laser surgical setting. (A) shows the usual positioning of the assistant and the nurse with the usual surgical instruments adopted during TOLMS; (B) and (C) shows the coupling system and the position of the exoscope during TOLMS with free-beam CO_2 laser in detail. In (D), the first surgeon moved the exoscope far from the surgical field to perform an endoscopic inspection; the exoscope can be returned to the saved surgical position by pushing a button.

the foot pedal and moving the joystick of the IMAGE1 PILOT to precisely align the surgical corridor perpendicular to the focal plane of the camera, and make laser delivery as orthogonal as possible (Fig. 4.4B and C). Moreover, the dedicated software is able to save the selected operating position by pushing together the foot pedal and the buttons 1 or 2 on the IMAGE1 PILOT. If the arm needs to be moved away (e.g., to better adjust the laryngeal exposure or to inspect the filed by an endoscope, Fig. 4.4D), the camera can be moved back to the saved position by pushing together the foot pedal and buttons 3 or 4, which are needed to adjust the position with fine remotely controlled movements.

4.3.2 Advantages and traps

The proposed transoral laser exoscopic setting is a feasible alternative to conventional TOLM. Patient selection follows the same rules applied to TOLM, through accurate endoscopic study of tumoral extension with preoperative flexible videoendoscopy and intraoperative evaluation with 0 degrees and 70 degrees telescopes. Radiological evaluation should be recommended if any suspicion of deep tissue involvement is presumed, or if the tumor is located in critical areas, such as a commissural one.

The main advantage of the exoscopic view is evident in academic institutions, where the possibility for assistants to follow the surgical procedure with the same 3D view of the main surgeon can make the learning curve potentially faster. Secondly, as recently observed, this surgical setting is fully suitable for the use of necessary personal protective equipment required for treatment of patients affected by air borne infection, such as COVID-19, including the use of face shields.[9,14]

The main limitation of the current exoscopic system equipped with a VITOM-3D camera, which should be considered as a relative contraindication compared to conventional TOLM, is related to the use of narrow laryngoscopes that are often employed for anterior commissure exposure that negatively influences the lighting of the surgical field.

4.3.3 Case reports

Herein we present two clinical cases in which the VITOM 3D-HD ARTip Cruise free-beam CO_2 laser setting was applied, underlining the details in terms of diagnostic evaluation and indications for this type of surgery.

4.3.3.1 Case 1: endoscopic supraglottic laryngectomy

A 55-year-old male, who was a smoker (20 pack/year) and drinker (2 AU/day) and affected by HIV infection without any other comorbidities, was referred to our institution. He had complained odynophagia, right otalgia, chronic cough, and dysphagia for a year with weight loss of 4 kg during the last 2 months. An ENT specialist at another center had already diagnosed a lesion of the laryngeal surface of the epiglottis, which was biopsy proven as squamous cell carcinoma. Evaluation at our department with videolaryngostroboscopy with a flexible ENF-V2 videoendoscope connected to an Evis Exera II CLV-180B light source (Visera Elite OTV-S190, Olympus Medical Systems Corporation, Tokyo, Japan) confirmed the presence of a cT2 supraglottic tumor involving the suprahyoid and infrahyoid laryngeal surface of the epiglottis (Fig. 4.5), not reaching the glottic plane nor infiltrating the preepiglottic space, as shown by the CT scan. The clinical case was discussed at a multidisciplinary tumor board, and an endoscopic surgical treatment associated with a staged bilateral neck dissection was planned.

The endoscopic surgical resection was performed by obtaining exposure of the larynx with a Hinni Distending Operating Laryngoscope (Karl Storz SE & Co. KG, Tuttlingen, Germany), allowing adequate exposure of the supraglottis and

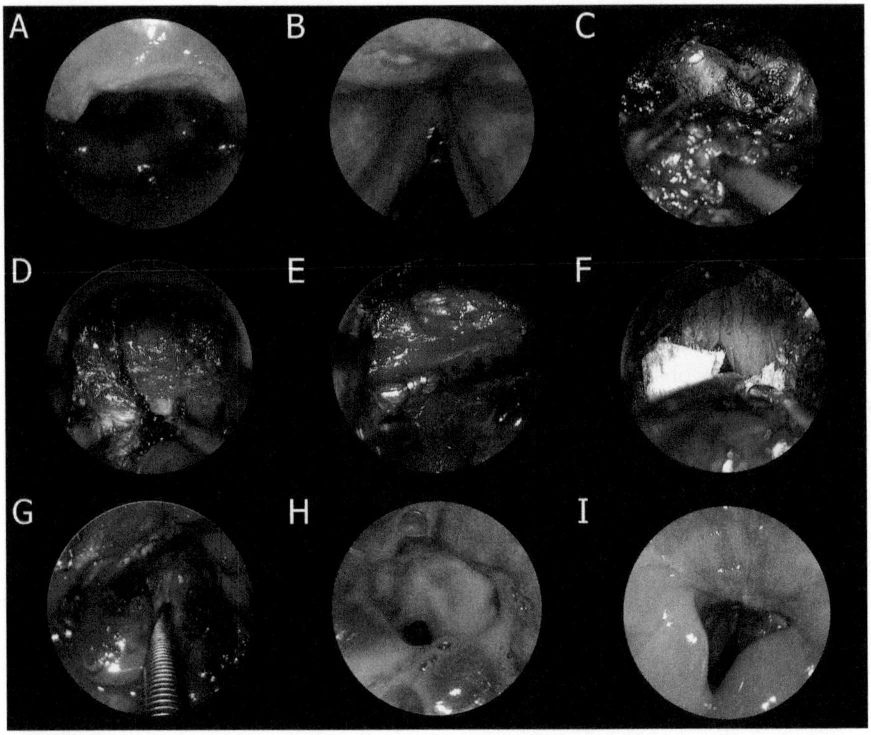

FIGURE 4.5

Clinical pictures of Case 1. (A, B) Pictures of the preoperative flexible videoendoscopy. (C) surgical view of the dissection along the subperichondral plane of the thyroid cartilage showing the second surgeon helping with the suction device; (D) identification of the epiglottic artery and its ligation (E). Surgical resection extending inferiorly to include the false vocal cords (F); the sponge helps to protect the true focal folds and gently manipulate the specimen; (G) shows intraoperative endoscopic evaluation at the end of the surgical procedure; the upper border of the thyroid cartilage is shown; (H) endoscopic evaluation 3 weeks after surgery; (I) final healing after 6 weeks.

positioning the superior blade inside the glossoepiglottic-vallecula. Intraoperative endoscopy with 0 degrees and 70 degrees telescopes confirmed the superficial extension of the tumor, which was confined to the entire laryngeal surface of the epiglottis without any further spreading toward its lingual surface, nor laterally to the aryepiglottic folds or inferiorly to the false vocal bands. Transoral resection was carried out with the VITOM 3D-HD held by the ARTip Cruise and coupled with the CO_2 laser micromanipulator for free-beam delivery. The resection performed was a medial supraglottic laryngectomy with resection of the preepiglottic space and ventricular bands (Type IIIb according to the European Laryngological Society classification[15]). The incision began by cutting the glossoepiglottic fold along the midline and along the valleculae until the hyoid bone was reached. To keep the entire preepiglottic space included in the specimen, the resection followed the thyrohyoid membrane reaching the upper border of the thyroid cartilage, and the inner surface of its lamina was exposed along a subperichondral plane reaching the anterior commissure. Bilaterally, the superior laryngeal arteries were clipped and the resection was performed along the aryepiglottic folds sparing the medial wall of the pyriform sinus to protect the airway. Inferiorly, both false vocal folds were included in the specimen to guarantee a safe inferior margin.

The surgical procedures, carried out with the exoscopic system, guaranteed a wider surgical space in front of the laryngoscope with beneficial assistance by the assistant surgeon using suction and pulling maneuvers, while having the same 3D view of the surgeon.

The final histopathological diagnosis confirmed a supraglottic squamous cell carcinoma (pT2), resected in free margins. One month later, after complete healing of the endolaryngeal wound, a bilateral selective neck dissection was performed including levels IIa—III—IV bilaterally, confirming the pT2N0 staging.

4.3.3.2 Case 2: endoscopic subligamental cordectomy

A 71-year-old male reported to our outpatient clinic referring the presence of a leucoplakia of the left oral commissure for several years, with presence of ulceration starting 1 month earlier. He referred smoking habit (50 pack/year) and frequent alcohol consumption (7.5 AU/day). His past medical history included therapy for hypertension and inguinal hernioplasty. Outpatient consultation was carried out by evaluating the upper aerodigestive tract with a flexible ENF-V2 videoendoscope and rigid telescope, integrated with high-definition television and NBI. Oral cavity endoscopic evaluation confirmed the presence of an erythroleukoplakia of the left oral commissure, without any vascular abnormalities inside the lesion nor around it and thickening at the digital palpation. Furthermore, videolaryngostroboscopy revealed a leucoplakia involving the midleft vocal cord. NBI did not show any vascular abnormalities and the mucosal wave was present as assessed by stroboscopy. The Laryngoscore was 1. Neck MRI confirmed a superficial mucosal lesion of the left buccal commissure without infiltration of the orbicularis oris muscle, while the glottic leukoplakia was not identifiable.

The surgical procedure encompassed transoral resection of the oral commissure lesion with primary closure and exoscopic CO_2 laser-assisted excisional biopsy of the glottic leukoplakia.

Laryngeal suspension was performed with a large bore laryngoscope (Microfrance Laryngoscopes 121, Medtronic ENT, Jacksonville, FL) that allowed clear visualization of the entire glottic plane with mild external counterpressure on the neck. Diagnostic evaluation was integrated by intraoperative endoscopy with rigid endoscopes (0 degrees and 70 degrees) with 4K white light and NBI evaluation, which confirmed the presence of a midcord leukoplakia of the left vocal cord (Fig. 4.6A and B) amenable to excisional biopsy by subepithelial or subligamental cordectomy (Type I or Type II, according to the ELS classification[16]). The VITOM

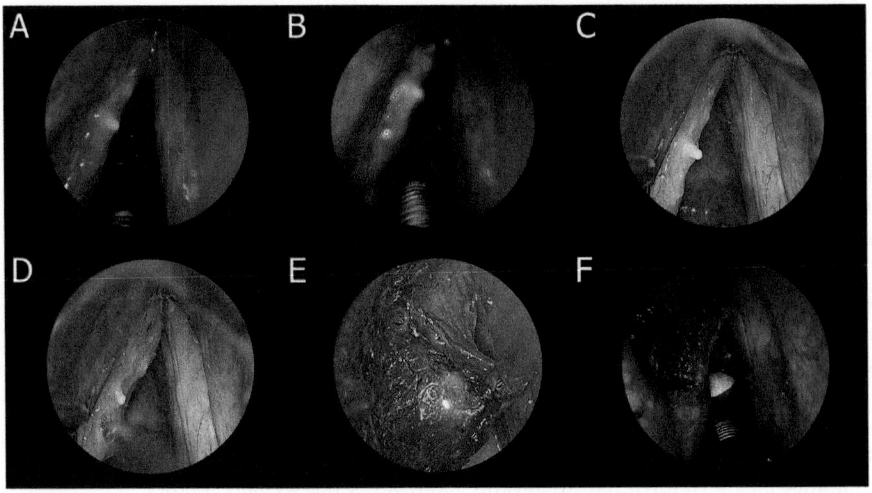

FIGURE 4.6

Clinical pictures of Case 2. (A, B) Endoscopic intraoperative view of the glottis showing a leukoplakia involving the midleft vocal cord, without any vascular abnormality detectable by NBI. Intraoperative view through the VITOM-3D in (C, D) shows saline infusion into Reinke's space with an incomplete hydrodissection, guiding a subligamental cordectomy (Type II), as shown in (E). (F) Endoscopic view of the surgical field at the end of the resection.

3D-HD hold by the ARTip Cruise and coupled with the CO_2 laser micromanipulator (Ultrapulse Laser CO_2, Lumenis, Yokneam, Israel) was positioned, and the entire surgical procedure was performed following the usual steps applied during conventional TOLM. Firstly, the mucoligamentous hydrodissection was tested with saline infusion into Reinke's space with an angled needle (Endocraft LLC, Boston, MA) to guide deep extension of the resection.[17] An incomplete hydrodissection was observed (Fig. 4.6C and D) thus guiding the choice toward subligamental cordectomy (Type II). The CO_2 laser procedure included a left ventriculectomy to better expose the surgical field. The superficial margins of the resection were defined without overcoming the anterior commissure to avoid undesired synechia, and the CO_2 resection was performed in a posterior to anterior direction cutting the vocal ligament that was included in the specimen, sparing the whole vocal muscle (Fig. 4.6E). The endoscopic view at the end of the surgical procedure is shown in Fig. 4.6F, and the histopathologic report was consistent with a high-grade dysplasia resected in free margins. The patient was submitted to endoscopic follow-up.

4.4 Future perspectives

Technical and technological advancements in the field of laryngeal surgery have helped to expand the indications for transoral minimally invasive conservative treatment, thus reducing complications and recurrence rates with a better control of surgical margins. This can be achieved thanks to more and more ergonomic and easy-to-use devices, among which the 3D-HD exoscopic systems have also brought the didactic potential to an entirely new level. Compared to traditional microscopic settings, this new concept appears to be more user-friendly and easily approachable, especially by unexperienced beginners, with a shorter learning curve.[18]

Additional research that improves the following issues will surely optimize the routine application of this system:

- Full integration of the micromanipulator with preset alignment and distance.
- Implementation of new technologies for laser control, such as the CALM concept setting[19] and stylus-based control.[20]
- Evolution of laryngoscopes and laryngeal suspension tools to minimize limitations in exposure.
- Quick and easy interchangeability between exoscopic and endoscopic settings and between CO_2 and fiber laser settings.

In light of this, progressive overlapping/substitution of the transoral robotic surgery (TORS) for supraglottic larynx and hypo- and oropharynx lesions, and the TOLM for glottic disease are desirable with the ultimate goal to overcome the limitations of conventional surgical techniques.

References

1. Crosetti E, Arrigoni G, Manca A, Caracciolo A, Bertotto I, Succo G. 3D exoscopic surgery (3Des) for transoral oropharyngectomy. *Front Oncol*. 2020;10:1–8. https://doi.org/10.3389/fonc.2020.00016.
2. De Virgilio A, Iocca O, Di Maio P, et al. Free flap microvascular anastomosis in head and neck reconstruction using a 4K three-dimensional exoscope system (VITOM 3D). *Int J Oral Maxillofac Surg*. 2020;49(9):1169–1173. https://doi.org/10.1016/j.ijom.2020.01.022.
3. Rubini A, Di Gioia S, Marchioni D. 3D exoscopic surgery of lateral skull base. *Eur Arch Otorhinolaryngol*. 2020;277(3):687–694. https://doi.org/10.1007/s00405-019-05736-7.
4. Smith S, Kozin ED, Kanumuri VV, et al. Initial experience with 3-dimensional exoscope-assisted transmastoid and lateral skull base surgery. *Otolaryngol Head Neck Surg*. 2019; 160(2):364–367. https://doi.org/10.1177/0194599818816965.
5. Oertel JM, Burkhardt BW. Vitom-3D for exoscopic neurosurgery: initial experience in cranial and spinal procedures. *World Neurosurg*. 2017;105:153–162. https://doi.org/10.1016/j.wneu.2017.05.109.
6. De Virgilio A, Costantino A, Ebm C, et al. High definition three-dimensional exoscope (VITOM 3D) for microsurgery training: a preliminary experience. *Eur Arch Otorhinolaryngol*. 2020;277(9):2589–2595. https://doi.org/10.1007/s00405-020-06014-7.

7. De Virgilio A, Costantino A, Mondello T, et al. Pre-clinical experience with the VITOM 3D and the ARTip Cruise system for micro-laryngeal surgery. *Laryngoscope*. 2021;131(1):136–138. https://doi.org/10.1002/lary.28675.
8. Carobbio ALC, Missale F, Fragale M, et al. Transoral laser microsurgery: feasibility of a new exoscopic HD-3D system coupled with free beam or fiber laser. *Lasers Med Sci*. 2021. https://doi.org/10.1007/s10103-020-03221-w.
9. Carobbio ALC, Filauro M, Parrinello G, Missale F, Peretti G. Microsurgical procedures during COVID-19 pandemic: the VITOM® 3D-HD exoscopic system as alternative to the operating microscope to properly use personal protective equipment (PPE). *Eur Arch Otorhinolaryngol*. 2020:1–4. https://doi.org/10.1007/s00405-020-06239-6.
10. Cosway B, Drinnan M, Paleri V. Narrow band imaging for the diagnosis of head and neck squamous cell carcinoma: a systematic review. *Head Neck*. 2016;38(Suppl 1):E2358–E2367. https://doi.org/10.1002/hed.24300.
11. Missale F, Carobbio A, Peretti G. The ORBEYE 4K 3D to safely replace selected microsurgical and transoral robotic procedures during COVID-19 pandemic. *Authorea*. 2020. https://doi.org/10.22541/au.158801242.22633679 (preprint).
12. Piazza C, Paderno A, Grazioli P, et al. Laryngeal exposure and margin status in glottic cancer treated by transoral laser microsurgery. *Laryngoscope*. May 2018;128(5):1146–1151. https://doi.org/10.1002/lary.26861.
13. Incandela F, Paderno A, Missale F, et al. Glottic exposure for transoral laser microsurgery: proposal of a mini-version of the laryngoscore. *Laryngoscope*. 2019;129(7):1617–1622. https://doi.org/10.1002/lary.27525.
14. Torretta S, Gaini LM, Pignataro L. Why Italian ENT physicians should be aware of SARS-CoV-2. *Acta Otorhinolaryngol Ital*. 2020;40(2):152–153. https://doi.org/10.14639/0392-100X-N0738.
15. Remacle M, Hantzakos A, Eckel H, et al. Endoscopic supraglottic laryngectomy: a proposal for a classification by the working committee on nomenclature, European Laryngological Society. *Eur Arch Otorhinolaryngol*. 2009;266(7):993–998. https://doi.org/10.1007/s00405-008-0901-8.
16. Remacle M, Eckel HE, Antonelli A, et al. Endoscopic cordectomy. A proposal for a classification by the Working Committee, European Laryngological Society. *Eur Arch Otorhinolaryngol*. 2000;257(4):227–231. https://doi.org/10.1007/s004050050228.
17. Mora F, Carta F, Missale F, et al. Laryngeal mid-cord erythroleukoplakias: how to modulate the transoral CO_2 laser excisional biopsy. *Cancers*. 2020;12(8):2165. https://doi.org/10.3390/cancers12082165.
18. Takahashi S, Toda M, Nishimoto M, et al. Pros and cons of using ORBEYE™ for microneurosurgery. *Clin Neurol Neurosurg*. 2018;174:57–62. https://doi.org/10.1016/j.clineuro.2018.09.010.
19. Deshpande N, Peretti G, Mora F, et al. Design and study of a next-generation computer-assisted system for transoral laser microsurgery. *OTO Open*. 2018;2(2). https://doi.org/10.1177/2473974X18773327.
20. Mattos LS, Caldwell DG, Peretti G, Mora F, Guastini L, Cingolani R. Microsurgery robots: addressing the needs of high-precision surgical interventions. *Swiss Med Wkly*. 2016;146:w14375. https://doi.org/10.4414/smw.2016.14375.

CHAPTER

Exoscope-assisted submandibular salivary stones surgery

5

Fabio Ferreli, MD [1,2], Matteo Di Bari, MD [1,2], Giovanni Colombo, MD [1,2]

[1]*Department of Biomedical Sciences, Humanitas University, Pieve Emanuele, Milan, Italy;*
[2]*Otorhinolaryngology Unit, IRCCS Humanitas Clinical and Research Center, Rozzano, Milan, Italy*

5.1 Historical background

Salivary stones were extracted as far as before Renascence, as well as abscesses and ranulas. With corpse dissection from the mid-17th century, the increasing anatomic and functional knowledge allowed to broaden surgical techniques.[1] In 1656, Thomas Wharton[2] was the first to describe the submandibular duct, in his paper "Adenographia," in which he described also the anatomy and function of salivary glands. In the same years, Marcello Malpighi[3] used pioneer microscopes to better understand salivary glands anatomy, with a structured point of view.

Concerning surgical tools and magnification, the microscope was used rarely and mostly for research and anatomical dissection purpose. From the late 19th century, surgical loupes were the main tool used by some surgeons to increase the magnification in this type of surgery.

Although surgical techniques have evolved over time, until 30 years ago, the main approach of Wharton's duct and oral pelvis surgery remained open transoral surgery. From the 1990s, there was an increasing attention to ductal lithiasis, with the development of minimally invasive and nonsurgical techniques of diagnosing and treating salivary gland duct stones, that evolved rapidly, in parallel to conventional surgery. Various combinations of diagnostic and treatment modalities were tried, such as endoscopes and dedicated endoscopic instruments, laser lithotriptors, and intra- or extracorporeal lithotripsy, with a proof of efficacy in most cases of ductal stones.

In 1991, Katz[4] published his early experience with a 0.8-mm mini-endoscope, revealing the endoscopic anatomy of the Wharton's duct. Later, in 1993, Katz and Koningsberger[5,6] reported independently their successful experience with endoscopic treatment of lithiasis.

Since then, enhanced optical resolution and miniaturization of instruments have resulted in the modern techniques of sialendoscopy. This modality provided a new tool to the surgeon, in addition to the removal of the entire salivary gland and to the marsupialization of the duct and removal of the stone.

Exoscope-Assisted Surgery in Otorhinolaryngology. https://doi.org/10.1016/B978-0-323-83168-0.00001-X

In 2015, Razavi et al.[7] described the robot-assisted sialolithotomy with sialendoscopy (RASS) for the management of large palpable hilar submandibular gland stones, as a safe and successful procedure, without damage to the lingual nerve.

The usefulness of 3D technology in improving surgical performance and accuracy was demonstrated in a recent 2019 study by Capaccio et al. describing the removal of submandibular stones with video-assisted transoral technique using 3D-HD sialendoscopy.[8]Recently, exoscope-assisted transoral removal of distal stone of the Wharton's duct was illustrated by our group.[9]

5.2 Introduction

Sialolithiasis is one of the most common nonneoplastic diseases of the salivary glands, with a 1.2% prevalence in the general population.[10] Submandibular glands account for about 79% of all salivary calculi; among these, 34% are localized in Wharton's duct, 57% in the hilum, and 9% inside the gland.[11] When the calculus blocks the salivary flow, symptoms may arise; swelling and pain of the submandibular gland, especially during mealtimes, or foreign body sensation in the floor of the mouth are the commonest reported. Beyond history taking and gland and mouth floor palpation, the main diagnostic tools are ultrasound scan or CT scan without contrast enhancement or diagnostic sialendoscopy. The first treatment indication can include the stimulation of the saliva production and the massage of the gland, to help getting smaller calculi to pass through the papilla. If calculi do not get removed spontaneously, the management is usually the surgical removal of the stone. Different approaches are available such as transoral removal of the calculi, sialoendoscopy, combined approach, or submandibular gland excision.

5.3 Principles

The well-known sialendoscope are semiflexible miniature endoscopes 0°, with integrated irrigatione and working channels, that guarantee adequate maneuverability through the delicate salivary ductal system and enable the minimally invasive removal of obstructions in the salivary ducts.

Although the sialendoscope has brought a paradigm shift in the management of parotid duct stones, especially on small stones, allowing direct removal of stone without risk on the facial nerve, Wharton's duct stones can be considered more challenging for many reasons.

The position of Wharton's duct punctum is quite variable, and it is not always easy to identify without any magnification. Surgical loupes are useful as they provide a good magnification for this anatomical site and they do not interfere with the surgical working space, but they affect just the view of the first surgeon.

Position and dimension of the stone are other factors that have to be taken into account. The majority of submandibular stones are hilar/anterior and result in difficulty to manage with sialendoscope alone, often requiring an intraoral incision for their removal. Sialoliths more than 3.5–4 mm are difficult to manage with a sialendoscope; they can either be broken down with extracorporeal shockwave lithotripsy or with laser fiber passed through the scope (intracorporeal lithotripsy), alternatively these larger stones can benefit from a combined approach (sialendoscope guided external approach).[12] For these manifold reasons, submandibular stone surgery can have a huge benefit from 3D exoscope; this innovative high definition rigid rod lens telescope can be suspended above the surgical field coming from the head of the patients and it produces high-quality full-HD three-dimensional images that can be visualized on a large-format HD 4K resolution flat screen by the surgeon and the other operating room personnel wearing 3D glasses. These features allow a shared high-detailed magnification that well assists the transoral removal of calculi.

The video tower system is the same as the sialendoscope, allowing fast and easy interchangeability between the two tools in combined procedures.

5.4 Indications and contraindications

The best suitable surgeries for exoscopic usage are a transoral approach to stones localized above the mylohyoid muscle in the anterior two-thirds of the floor of the mouth, irrelevant of their palpability. The indication of exoscope-assisted transoral calculus removal can be extended to transoral submandibulotomy when calculi are identified by palpation and sonography and localized in the posterior part of the floor of the mouth.[11]

A relative contraindication of exoscope usage is deep hilar and intraparenchymal stones in the Wharton's duct, in which endoscopy-assisted transoral removal has to be preferred,[13] but if the calculus is more than 3.5–4 mm a combined sialendoscope-exoscope approach can be feasible.

Contraindication to surgery, in general, is the acute inflammatory stage.

5.5 Operating room organization

Our operating room layout was conceived to allow two surgeons to work closely and to permit the surgical nurse to have a free range of movement to help the surgeons (Fig. 5.1). An adequate working space is mandatory to ensure maximum efficiency and an easy access to all resources.

The patient lies supine on an electrically operated surgical table, with the head as close as possible to the superior edge of the table. The patient has to be strapped into the final desired position. Position adjustments needed prior or during surgery would be achieved with the inclination of the operating room (OR) table, controlled by the OR nurse with the remote control, positioned at the foot of the table.

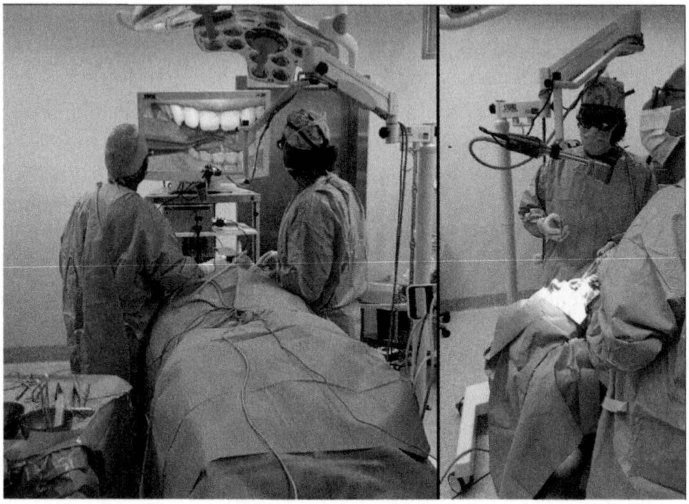

FIGURE 5.1

Operating room layout and 3D exoscope position.

The anesthetist, the anesthesia nurse, and all the anesthesia equipment are settled at the table foot. If a general anesthesia is performed, the endotracheal tube is secured to the mouth edge and to the patient's chest and is directed to the bed foot as well as the intravenous and other lines.

The surgeon and the assistant stand on each side of the patient's head. The scrub nurse stands behind the first surgeon, with the Mayo stand that can be placed over the surgical table. The surgeon and all the operating room personnel have to wear 3D glasses to be involved in the surgery.

The video tower with the 3D 4k monitor has to be positioned at the top of the surgical bed; with this positioning, all operating room personnel can share the same view on the same monitor. One or more supplementary 2D or 3D monitors can be placed if necessary, increasing the possibility of sharing, for example when there are multiple observers.

The observer can have a proper place behind the surgeon or at the feet of the table, without interfering with the surgical act, but instead sharing the same view of the first surgeon on the same monitor or a proper settled additional one. A shared vision is crucial for teaching, and the 3D technology allows also the same depth perception, with a high involvement in the surgery.

5.6 Exoscope positioning

The 3D exoscope is positioned with the base on the opposite side of the first surgeon, behind the assistant. The flexible layout of the holding system allows an easy and precise positioning of the camera without obstructing the monitor view (Fig. 5.1).

The second cantilever arm and the smaller "L" that holds the camera have to enter over the surgical field from the top of the table side, at the head of the patient with the camera over the surgical field in between the two surgeons. The camera is properly oriented toward the patient oral cavity, in a vertical asset. In this type of surgery, the operative distance can be also a bit more than the conventional 20 cm, at the level of the surgeon's shoulder; in this way, surgeon movements are not affected at all and a high-quality magnification can still be achieved.

Once the exoscope has been settled in his desired position, then it should be partially blocked, to not allow open-range motions but controlled movements. After the ceiling and the surgeon's positioning, the camera head can be easily reached by both surgeons, for every movement and adjustment during surgery, even with a single hand.

Zoom (2–16 magnification), focusing, and other functions are controlled through a Pilot controller that can be fixed on the operating table and positioned near the hand of the surgeon or of the assistant through its smallholding arm. The pilot can also be controlled by another assistant, especially a trainee; it is really intuitive, and it increases the attention and the involvement in the surgery.

5.7 Surgical technique

Distal stones in the Wharton's duct are the best suitable for approaching exoscope-assisted transoral removal of sialolith, and the exoscope can be used for all operative steps.[14,15]

Intraoral disinfection can be done with a betadine-soaked cotton ball. After disinfection, the oral cavity can be thoroughly washed with sterile saline. In our experience, we perform the surgery in local anesthesia in the operating room, with 2% lidocaine with 1:100,000 epinephrine. The injection can be performed on the floor of the mouth (Fig. 5.2A).

Through the pilot control, an adequate magnification of the oral pelvis can be obtained, and, after adjusting the focus, the distal stone can be well visualized, as well as the profile of the Wharton's duct (Fig. 5.2B).

A 1-cm incision can be made at the entrance of the duct, at the level of the stone (Fig. 5.2C).

Then, blunt dissection to the Wharton's duct can be performed, and then it can be incised right under the calculus. The calculus can then be easily tilted out (Fig. 5.3A).

No further dissection is needed to identify the lingual nerve when the calculus is in such a position and no other lithiasic formations are identified at preoperative imaging. Considering that the lingual nerve runs below the Wharton's duct, a large, palpable calculus would also provide protection to the nerve.

The entrance of the submandibular gland's duct is easily confirmed through the 3D 4K Vitom systems (Fig. 5.3B). Then, the duct has to be washed with a saline and steroid solution.

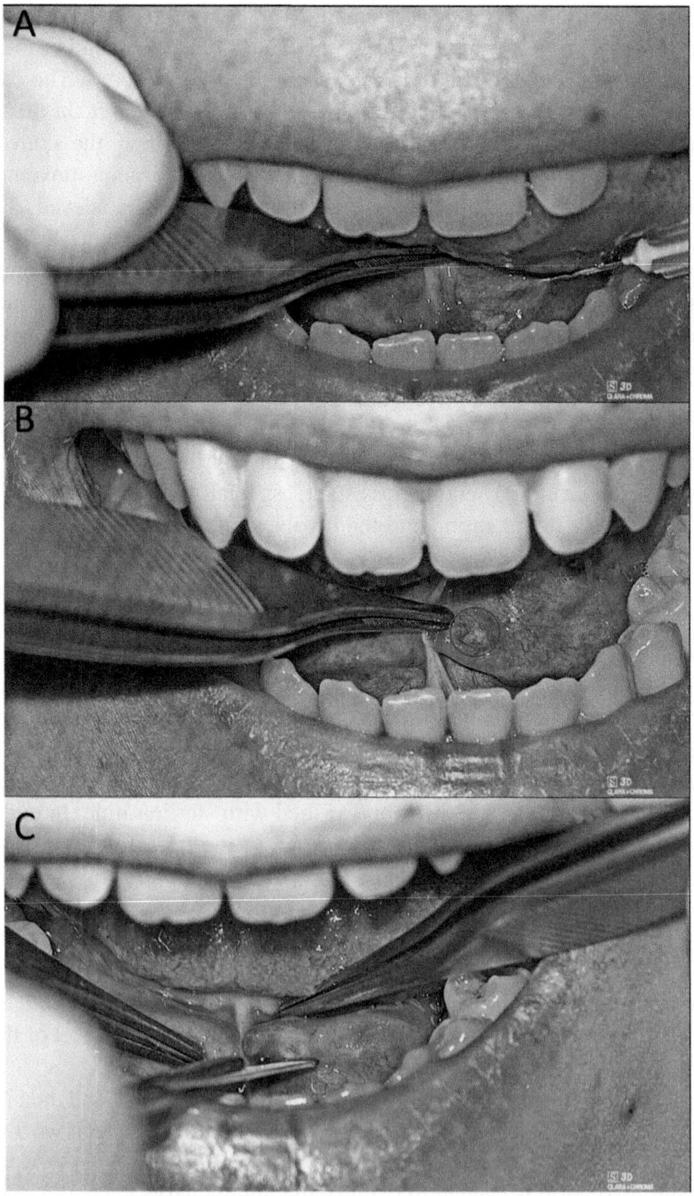

FIGURE 5.2

(A) Local anesthesia administration on the floor of the mouth. (B) Magnification of the floor of the mouth obtained through the exoscope (VITOM 3D, Karl Storz), with the evidence of distal stone in the left Wharton's duct. (C) Incision.

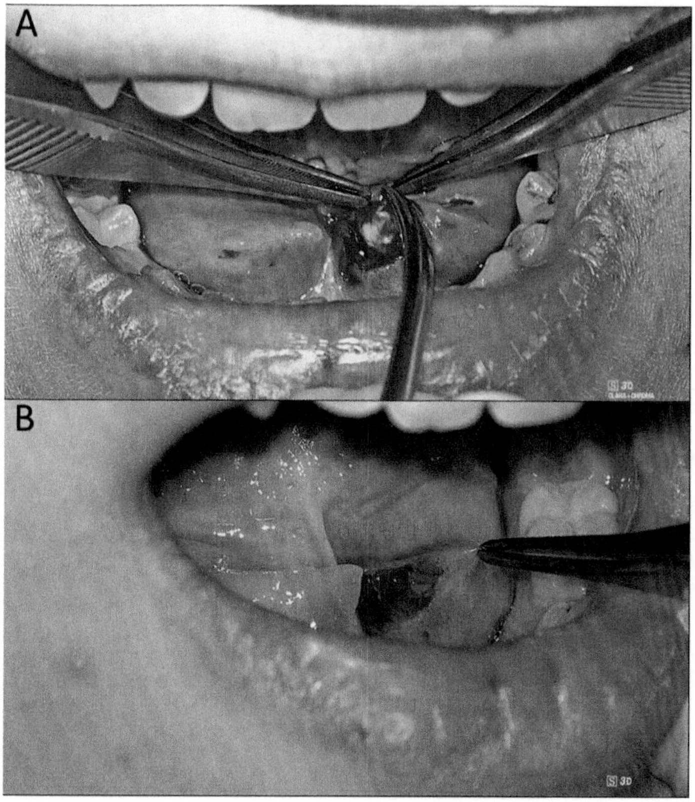

FIGURE 5.3

(A) Isolation of the calculus in the Wharton's duct. (B) Lumen of the left submandibular gland's duct.

An angiocatheter of the proper size, usually 20G, can carefully be inserted and fixed with a suture (Fig. 5.4A and B). The incision stays open without the need for sialodochoplasty.[16,17]

The patient can be discharged within the same day. After 3 days, the angiocatheter can be removed, and usually within a week, the patient develops a neo-ostium near the papilla.

This exoscope-assisted approach can be even more advantageous during the particular situation, such as when the calculus is very difficult to reach, because it has a more posterior location or when it is partially plunged beneath the mylohyoid muscle, and the surrounding anatomical structures may not be well visualized, with a greater risk of surgical damage. In these cases, a 3D exoscope can allow a high-detailed magnification and better visualization of the oral floor and therefore minimizing the risk of lingual nerve injury. Further experience is needed in such calculi. The dissection of the lingual nerve exoscope-assisted should be considered if the preoperative ultrasound shows a large calculus located posteriorly or beneath the mylohyoid muscle.

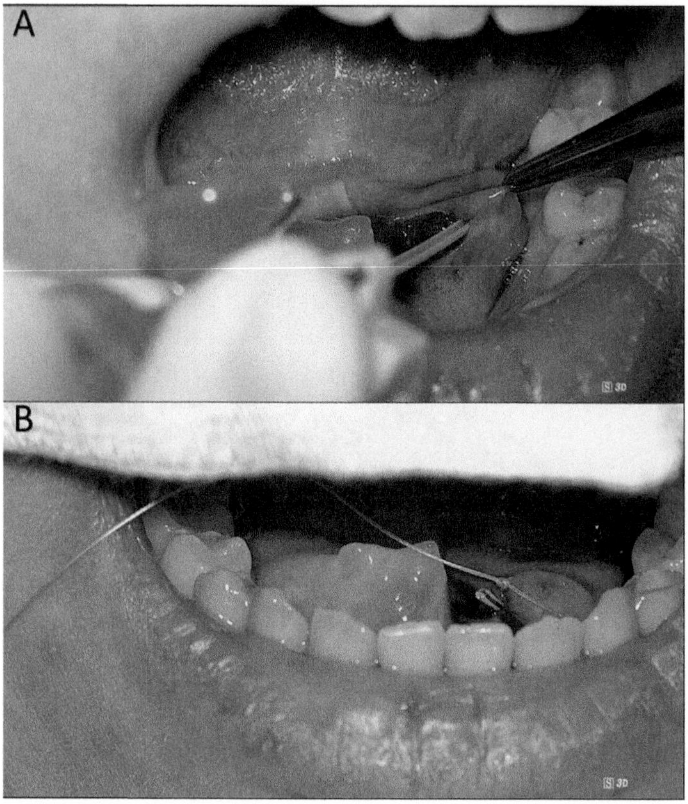

FIGURE 5.4

(A) Angiocatheter (20G) insertion in the left submandibular gland's duct. (B) Angiocatheter (20G) inserted in the left submandibular gland's duct and fixed with a suture.

5.8 Conclusions

The exoscope represents a valid tool for transoral removal of calculi, which is the gold standard for hilar/anterior stone, and it can allow a precise surgical dissection of the oral floor, thus reducing the risks for iatrogenic lesion of the lingual nerve in more distal stone. Moreover, it showed a high potential for training and educational purposes.

Furthermore, the exoscope shares the advantages of lightness, maneuverability, and compactness with the sialendoscope, allowing for highly accurate minimally invasive surgery. The sialendoscope, which is effective as a standalone treatment tool in small proximal stones, can benefit from a combined use with the exoscope to identify the punctum of the Wharton duct. This combined procedure is made easier by the sharing of the same video column.

5.9 Pearls and pitfalls

- A proper positioning of video tower system, exoscope, and surgeons is essential for access the oral cavity
- Distal stones in the Wharton's duct are the best suitable for exoscope-assisted transoral approach
- The 3D Exoscope can be used for all operative steps, and it allows a precise visualization and manipulation of the Wharton's duct and the calculus
- The exoscopic video tower system is the same as the sialendoscope, allowing fast and easy interchangeability between the two tools in combined procedures.
- Sialendoscopy has to be preferred in deep hilar and intraparenchymal stones removal.

References

1. Melo GM, Cervantes O, Abrahao M, Covolan L, Ferreira ES, Baptista HA. A brief history of salivary gland surgery. *Rev Col Bras Cir.* 2017;44(4):403–412.
2. Cook HJ. Thomas Wharton's Adenographia, first published in London in 1656. *Med Hist.* 1998;42(3):411–412.
3. Malpighi M. *Opera Omnia.* Londini: Prostant apud Robertum Scott; 1686.
4. Katz PH. Endoscopie des glands salivaries. *Ann Radiol.* 1991;34:110–113.
5. Katz PH. Traitement endoscopique des lithiasis salivares. *J Otorhinolaryngol.* 1993;42: 33–36.
6. Konigsberger R, Feyh J, Goetz, et al. Endoscopically-controlled electrohydraulic intracorporeal shock wave lithotripsy (EISL) of salivary stones. *J Otorhinolaryngol.* 1993; 22:12–13.
7. Razavi C, Pascheles C, Samara G, Marzouk M. Robot-assisted sialolithotomy with sialendoscopy for the management of large submandibular gland stones. *Laryngoscope.* 2016;126(2):345–351.
8. Capaccio P, Di Pasquale D, Bresciani L, Torretta S, Pignataro L. 3D video-assisted transoral removal of deep hilo-parenchymal sub-mandibular stones. *Acta Otorhinolaryngol Ital.* 2019;39(6):367–373.
9. Ferreli F, Di Bari M, Mercante G, De Virgilio A, Spriano G. 3D 4K VITOM-assisted transoral removal of distal stone in the Wharton's duct. *Am J Otolaryngol.* 2020: 102821. https://doi.org/10.1016/j.amjoto.2020.102821.
10. Rauch S, Gorlin RJ. Diseases of the salivary glands. In: Gorlin RJ, Goldman HM, eds. *Oral Pathology.* 6th ed. St. Louis: Mosby; 1970:997–1003.
11. Zenk J, Constantinidis J, Al-Kadah B, Iro H. Transoral removal of submandibular stones. *Arch Otolaryngol Head Neck Surg.* 2001;127(4):432–436.
12. Singh PP, Gupta V. Sialendoscopy: introduction, indications and technique. *Indian J Otolaryngol Head Neck Surg.* 2014;66(1):74–78.
13. Zhao YN, Zhang YQ, Ye X, Meng Y, Xie XY, Liu DG. Endoscopy-assisted transoral removal of deep hilar and intraparenchymal stones in the Wharton's duct. *Chin J Stomatol.* 2018;53(12):826–831.

14. Juul ML, Wagner N. Objective and subjective outcome in 42 patients after treatment of sialolithiasis by transoral incision of Wharton's duct: a retrospective middle-term follow-up study. *Eur Arch Otorhinolaryngol*. 2014;271(11):3059–3066.
15. Capaccio P, Clemente IA, McGurk M, Bossi A, Pignataro L. Transoral removal of hilo-parenchymal submandibular calculi: a long-term clinical experience. *Eur Arch Otorhinolaryngol*. 2011;268(7):1081–1086.
16. Park JH, Kim JW, Lee YM, Oh CW, Chang HS, Lee SW. Long-term study of sialodochoplasty for preventing submandibular sialolithiasis recurrence. *Clin Exp Otorhinolaryngol*. 2012;5(1):34–38.
17. Woo SH, Kwon MS, Park JJ, Kim JP. Anatomical study of the submandibular gland duct after removal of a distal stone without sialodochoplasty: a sialographic evaluation of a clinical phase II trial. *Br J Oral Maxillofac Surg*. 2016;54(5):556–560.

CHAPTER

Exoscope-assisted oropharyngeal surgery

6

Giovanni Succo, MD, PhD [1,2], Erika Crosetti, MD, PhD [1]

[1]*Head and Neck Oncology Unit, Candiolo Cancer Institute, FPO – IRCCS, Candiolo, Turin, Italy;*
[2]*Department of Oncology, University of Turin, Orbassano, Turin, Italy*

6.1 Introduction

The oropharynx is currently one of the most affected sites in head and neck oncology. Over the past 20 years, the incidence of oropharyngeal cancer has increased significantly, especially in younger people. This trend is clearly related to previous human papillomavirus infection.[1–5]

For advanced-stage oropharyngeal cancer, treatment generally includes at least two therapeutic modalities (surgery followed by radiation therapy or concurrent chemoradiotherapy), whereas for early disease treatment consists of surgery or radiation therapy alone. Radical surgery is particularly challenging because the oropharynx is involved in the crucial functions of swallowing, breathing, and speech, therefore early-stage cancers are frequently treated by radiation therapy alone.[6]

Historically, oncologic oropharyngeal surgery has been limited to open approaches (lateral pharyngotomy, pull-through, transmandibular approach), allowing excellent direct access to the disease, resulting in considerable functional and aesthetic sequelae. Therefore, nonsurgical organ preservation therapeutic options have progressively gained ground over time, guaranteeing similar oncological results, net of less invasiveness, and reduction of the impact on quality of life.

Following an initial enthusiastic spell, treatments based on chemoradiation protocols also demonstrated a significant rate of long-term dysfunctional sequelae, in turn extremely debilitating with a worsening of perceived quality of life. There was therefore a need to improve the options for surgical treatment allowing oncological and functional results similar to nonsurgical options to be obtained and minimizing the morbidity and the burden of treatments. This led to the development of minimally invasive transoral surgical techniques, such as laser and robotic surgery.

The recent introduction of 3D exoscopic surgery introduced interesting technical improvements in head and neck surgery, especially in transoral surgery, with the aims of replacing robotic surgery and minimizing the costs of the procedures.

In 2020, we have coined the term 3Dees (3D exoscopic/endoscopic surgery) to describe the use of the 3D VITOM Exoscope System/3D optics (Karl Storz, Tuttlingen, Germany) for the treatment of tumors of the oropharynx and oral cavity at an

Exoscope-Assisted Surgery in Otorhinolaryngology. https://doi.org/10.1016/B978-0-323-83168-0.00009-4

early-intermediate stage and to treat benign pathologies. Our aim has been to develop and rejuvenate the traditional transoral surgical technique with the addition of 3D screen vision, to analyze the efficacy and safety of the surgical procedures, and to test the system's ability in terms of surgical precision and shared surgical vision in comparison to transoral robotic surgery (TORS).

6.2 History

In 1951, Huet first described the transoral lateral oropharyngectomy (TLO) procedure for treating early invasive squamous cell carcinoma (SCC) of the tonsillar region.[7] TLO was reported to be an effective treatment option with safe oncologic outcomes for tumors of the lateral oropharyngeal wall, and it could represent an alternative to traditional aggressive surgical procedures, such as the transmandibular or transpharyngeal approaches.[8]

Lacourreye et al. reported 5-year local control rates of 89%−89.6% and 81.7%−85.8% in T1 and T2 oropharyngeal cancer treated with TLO, respectively. Moreover, other Authors reported 80% local control rate for selected oropharyngeal T3 and T4a.[9,10] Nevertheless, Huet's procedure did not achieve widespread acceptance among head and neck surgeons due to the narrow surgical field, which was difficult to reach because the first surgeon's view was limited (many tonsil and pharyngeal cancers are difficult or impossible to reach through the mouth under direct vision), and the poor maneuverability of surgical instruments.

In 2003, Steiner[11] attempted to overcome the drawbacks shown by TLO by introducing the use of microscope and transoral laser microsurgery (TLM) for the resection of oropharyngeal tumors, giving the surgeon better magnification and illumination of the surgical field. Although this was a significant improvement in transoral surgery allowing surgeons access to oropharyngeal sites that were hard to reach without an open approach, the microscope does not allow viewing around corners (it cannot be rotated along three-dimensional axes) while the 3D view is restricted to the first operator. In addition, it is only possible to execute straight/tangential cutting lines with the CO_2 laser, limiting the ability to make angled cuts around bulky structures or tumors.

To improve the efficacy of transoral access able to avoid the limitations of TLM, surgeons investigated the potential of surgical robotic platforms. TORS was performed for the first time in 2005 by Hockstein and colleagues,[12,13] while the earliest series of outcomes were published later by Weinstein, O'Malley, and colleagues.[14,15]

In recent years, several studies have shown that TORS may be an effective alternative to open surgery.[16–27] The high-resolution, magnified three-dimensional view of the operative field provided by TORS allows excellent visualization of the target area. Many other advantages have been highlighted: stable three-dimensional binocular magnification allowing "en bloc" resection to be performed with better identification of nerves and vessels; motion scaling; tremor filtration; a shortened learning curve and superior ergonomics for the surgeon. Moreover, surgery-associated morbidity is reduced with the robotic technique, improving functional outcomes compared to open approaches, and length of hospitalization is also reduced.

However, TORS faces some obstacles in pharyngeal and laryngeal surgery because the introduction of the robotic arms and instruments into narrow cavities can be difficult. Tumor exposure can be inadequate and can interfere with the robotic arms, and airway management can be challenging. In addition, the surgeon does not experience any intraoperative tactile feedback with this approach. Finally, robot-assisted surgery is costly with great obstacles to widespread uptake of this surgical option. Not all institutions have Da Vinci robotic platforms (Intuitive Surgical, Sunnyvale, CA), and there is often competition for the system among different specialties. Most hospitals cannot afford to purchase such an expensive device, particularly in developing countries.

6.3 3D exoscopic surgery by VITOM

Based on these considerations and keeping in mind that the oropharynx is easily accessible using a conventional surgical approach and that there may also be benefits from tactile feedback from the lesion, the introduction of the 3D VITOM Exoscope System has progressively spread. The aim is to improve surgical vision during the entire surgical procedure, and to reduced costs compared to robotic surgery when this approach is used.

Applied first in neurosurgery,[28,29] urology, and gynecologic surgery,[30] the use of VITOM is now starting to increase in ENT surgery as well. At present, only a few series have been reported in the Literature.[31,32]

6.4 Surgical procedure

6.4.1 Selection of patients

This is crucial in all types of transoral surgical procedures. Three categories should be considered when evaluating transoral candidacy: anatomic limits, patient comorbidities, and cancer characteristics. It is imperative to consider that unfavorable anatomy can impair adequate access and the view of the surgical field. Specific anatomic conditions could limit the exoscopic approach (reduced mandibular width, trismus with mouth opening <1.5 cm). Other anatomic restrictions, such as retrognathia and cervical spine inflexibility, do not represent an absolute contraindication to the use of VITOM as they are in robotic procedures. It is important to measure inter-incisive distance to estimate the ability of the transoral approach, and to provide good lesion exposure.

In any case, if the extent of exposure does not result optimal to guarantee adequate oncological radicality, open approaches or non-surgical treatments should be considered.

6.4.2 Operating room setting

The patient is placed in a supine position without any interscapular support. The procedures are carried out under general anesthesia, performed with nasopharyngeal intubation or by tracheostomy with intubation. For the execution of lateral oropharyngectomy, the 90 degrees VITOM is assembled on a mechanical holder and with an autostatic arm attached to the bed at a distance of about 35−40 cm from the patient's mouth, along the visual axis between the surgeon's eye and the operative target, so replacing the vision of the whole surgical team. A sterile cover is then draped over the system. Using this holder, the exoscope is not easy to place and move. At this time, this is a weak point of the technique, that makes maneuvering and the disposition of the right operative setting less fluid. More recently, a latest-generation robotic holder (ARTip *cruise*) has been successfully proposed for VITOM.

The main 3D monitor (55 in.) is placed beside the operating table directly in front of the first surgeon, while a secondary 3D monitor is oriented in front of the assistant. An intuitive control unit with a 3D wheel (joystick) is used to control the camera, with four programmable function keys. Surgery is more comfortable when performed by three surgeons, but it is always possible for the first or second surgeon to adjust the controller as it is covered with a sterile coating, or where not covered, it can be maneuvered by other members of the surgical team not working directly in the operating field. A joystick (IMAGE1 PILOT) can also be attached to a holding system to be controlled directly by the first surgeon when needed.

The surgeon is positioned at the patient's head, facing the main monitor. The first assistant sits on the left/right of the surgeon (depending on the side of the lesion) and, during the procedure, helps using retractors, Yankauer suction tube, bipolar cautery, and by positioning vascular clips. The second assistant sits on the opposite side, using the controller (IMAGE1 PILOT) covered with a sterile coating, and maintaining the focus of the camera on the surgical field, adjusting the optical magnification, and applying different camera enhancing tools (Storz Professional Image Enhancement System (SPIES)). The scrub nurse stays behind the surgeon. All operators wear 3D passive-polarized glasses (Fig. 6.1).

To improve visualization of the base of the tongue and supraglottis, the VITOM can also be replaced by TIPCAM (Karl Storz), a 3D laparoscopic video endoscope (0 degrees or 30 degrees), 10 mm in diameter. TIPCAM benefits from well-known visualization modes for diagnosis and therapy with clearer differentiation of tissue structures (CLARA, CHROMA, and SPECTRA visualization modes) (Fig. 6.2).

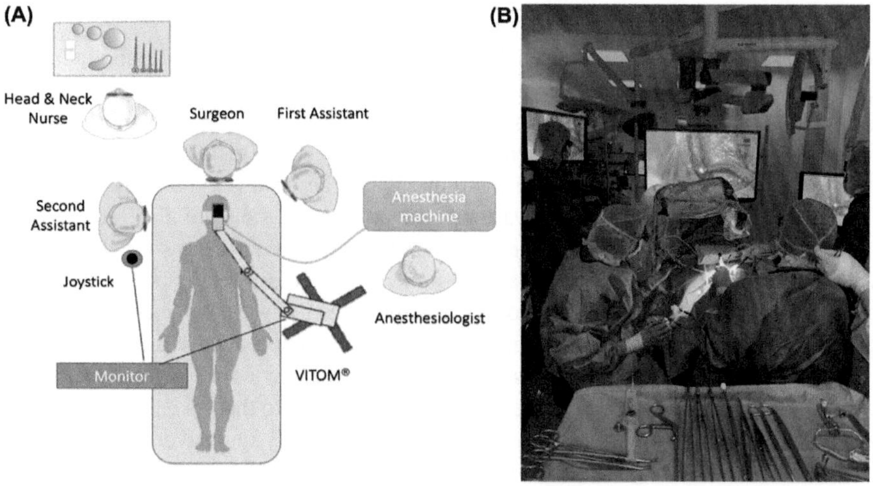

FIGURE 6.1

(A) Operating room setting with VITOM (scheme). (B) Operating room setting with VITOM (live surgery).

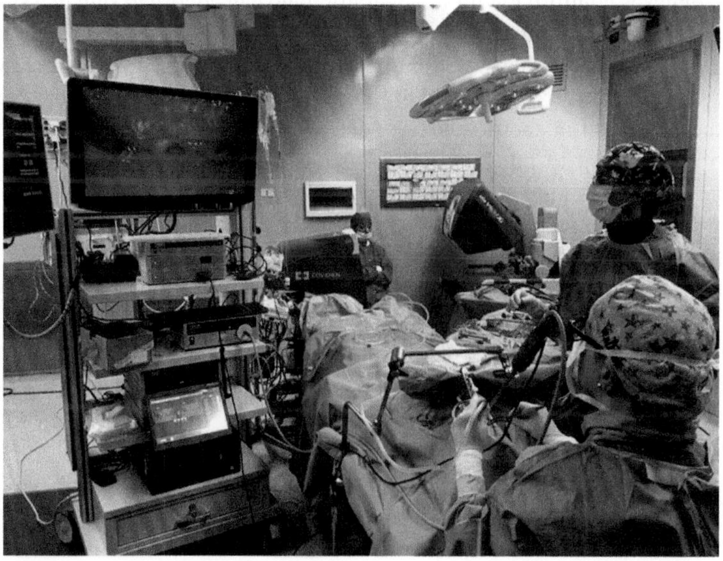

FIGURE 6.2

Operating room setting with TIPCAM (live surgery).

6.4.3 Surgical technique

A comfortable transoral exposure of the lesion is sought to visualize its boundaries completely and to have sufficient space to manipulate the surgical instruments. Different types of mouth retractors can be used. Surgical instruments should be at least 24 cm long (from 24 to 30 cm) because of the depth of the structures to be reached. Different kinds of cutting instruments can be used (bipolar scissors, CO_2 fiber laser, ultrasound tools), and various types of angled tools are also required.

When using the CO_2 fiber laser, it is mandatory to cover the nasotracheal tube with a wet swab or to use specifically designed tubes to avoid any possible fire in the airways. In any case, it is important to communicate with the anesthesiologist to reduce FiO_2 below 30% to prevent this eventuality, before using cautery or laser.

The characteristics of the 3Dees images are comparable to those of the operating microscope and the 3D optics of the Da Vinci system, due to their excellent ability to provide 3D visual information, that is used to interactively maneuver the exoscope camera. Other advantages are the depth of field, magnification, and image contrast and color, allowing effective manipulation of the anatomic structures. The most advantageous aspects are represented by the magnification of the anatomic details: the vascularization and irregularities of the mucosa are perfectly visible. The 3Dees provide a wide working space, and it is extremely useful for training and educational purposes. Both images and video sequences can be stored digitally.

Ergonomics is comfortable for the operator, who can choose to stay in a sitting or standing position, having the screen in front at the same height. Surgery performed with a 3D screen is not bothersome for operators, even for longer procedures, as long as the screen is placed frontally, and at the same height as the operator's eyes.

For the execution of the procedures, conventional surgical instruments can be used (no requirement to purchase other instruments), and this is undoubtedly an advantage in terms of immediacy, simplicity of use and low cost. Other hemostatic tools can be safely used (Focus, LigaSure, Thunderbeat, flexible CO_2 fiber laser, etc.) with complete visual control (Fig. 6.3).

We have applied the 3Dees approach for transoral resection of oropharyngeal SCC,[33] with or without neck dissection and reconstruction with free flaps. In our experience, most transoral surgical procedures enjoy the same benefits as provided by TORS, in terms of lower morbidity, fewer complications, and faster local healing and rehabilitation (Fig. 6.4).

Setup of 3Dees is easy and intuitive. This technique allows transoral surgery to be performed with indirect but straight visualization/magnification for the whole surgical team, and the team members are able to work with greater precision. Moreover, the exoscope allows the direct maneuverability of instruments providing a tactile sensibility, impossible to achieve when operating by TORS.

The 3Dees approach can also have immediate and straightforward application in non oncologic surgical procedures (tonsillectomy, lateral pharyngoplasty, etc.) (Fig. 6.5). During reconstruction, the approach can be useful while insetting a free flap in the oral cavity/oropharynx without opening the mandible, since the

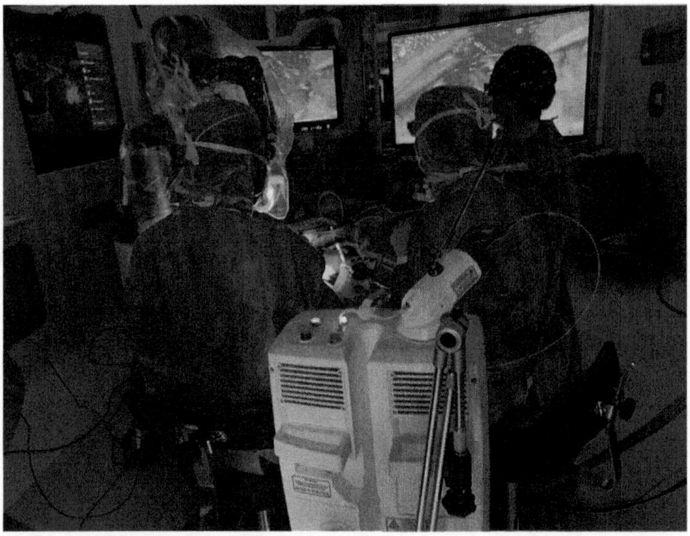

FIGURE 6.3

Operating room setting with VITOM and flexible CO_2 fiber laser (live surgery).

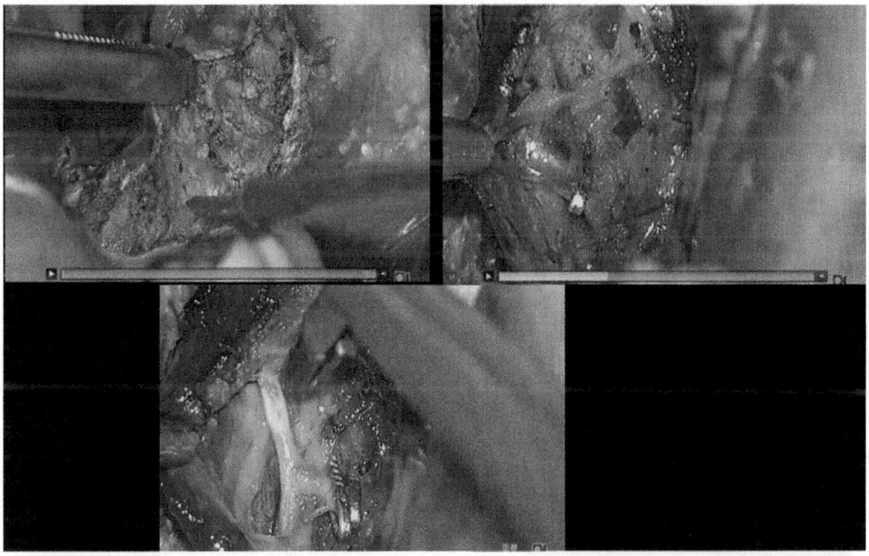

FIGURE 6.4

Transoral resection of oropharyngeal squamous cell carcinoma with VITOM.

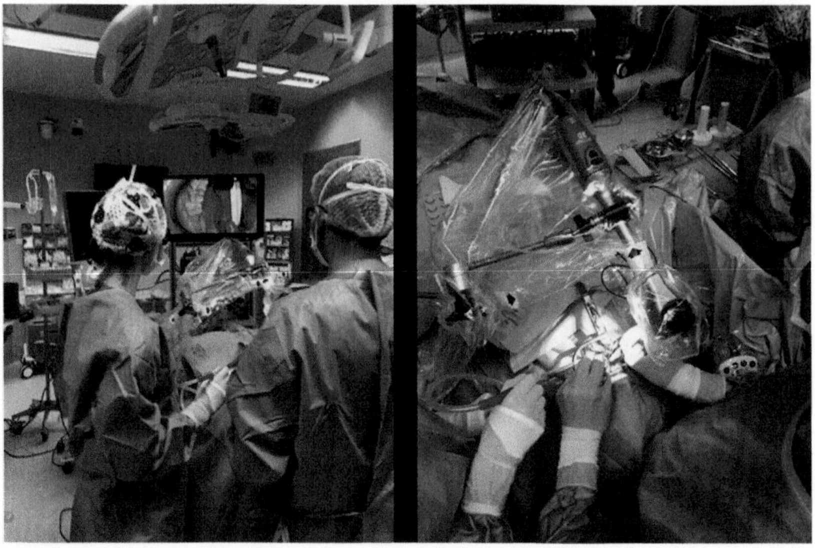

FIGURE 6.5

Operating room setting with VITOM in lateral pharyngoplasty surgical procedure.

vision provided by the exoscope facilitates transoral suturing of the flap to the mucosa. The combination of enhanced vision and use of a barbed suture is helpful in reducing operating time and fistula rate (Fig. 6.6).

Furthermore, the 3D exoscope permits a careful endoscopic work-up, which is useful in checking the correct surgical field exposure and in completing a good

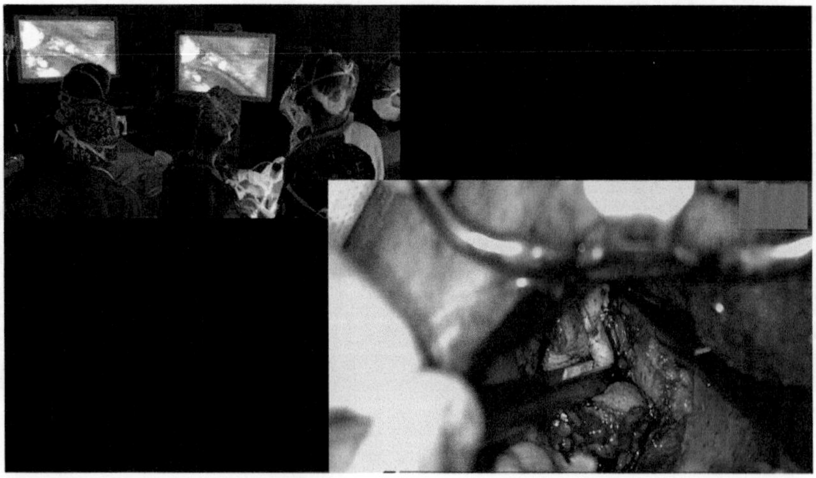

FIGURE 6.6

Operating room setting with VITOM in forearm free flap insetting and suturing.

and safe resection by TORS. A well-executed work-up can also save time during setting up for robotic surgery, for example, by assessing beforehand which self-retaining retractor to use (Fig. 6.7).

Finally, 3Dees is extremely beneficial in the learning process, especially for residents, fellows, students, and OR staff, thanks to the shared visual experience available to all operators, and always with wide high-resolution screens.

3Dees can guide the trainees' surgical maneuvers, and thus they may gain confidence in navigating the anatomic structures and in performing microsurgical techniques while watching directly on the 3D screen. The inside-out anatomic study and the indispensable knowledge for surgeons who undertake transoral surgery of the oropharynx are facilitated by the 3Dees approach, for both the fidelity of vision and equipment logistics that makes it more easily transportable in the cadaver lab than the robotic platform. Moreover, the possibility to record in high definition enables the surgeons to share videos for didactic sessions, meetings, and courses on surgical techniques.

At present, in a health policy aimed at reducing costs, it is difficult to have up-to-date technologies. The cost of the exoscopic platform is similar to that of an operating microscope with an electromagnetic brake holder and is about 10 times, lower than the Da Vinci robotic platform. The cost of disposable equipment for each surgical procedure is about 40–60 dollars, composed of two sterile sheaths for the holder and controller. Even the price of maintenance is considerably lower.

The current drawbacks can be represented by the mechanical holder that is not always comfortable to move during surgery, and the necessity to wear 3D glasses for a prolonged period that can lead to headaches and nasal pain (in only two patients out of 41 in our experience).

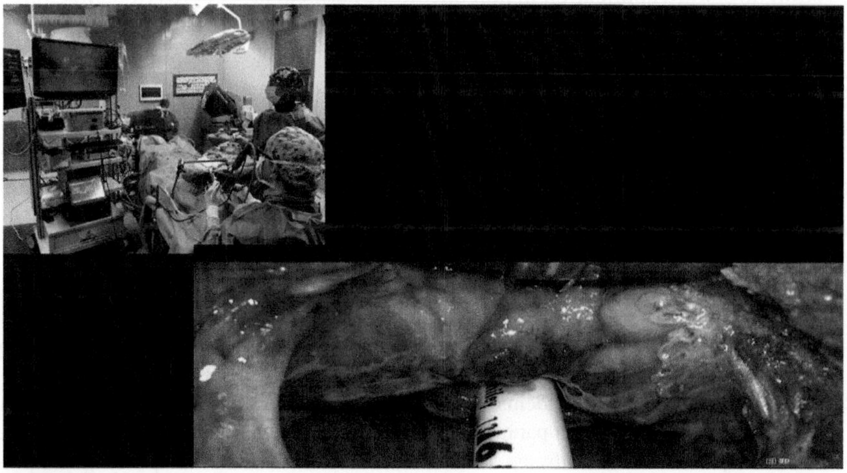

FIGURE 6.7

Operating room setting with TIPCAM in endoscopic work-up for base of tongue squamous cell carcinoma (BOT SCC).

With the introduction of any new surgical approach, it is common to face difficulties achieving the optimum layout of the operating room, and the most favorable position for the exoscope/holder/camera control wheel (joystick) in the surgical field. However, the level of fine operativity achievable by TORS during dissection in the parapharyngeal space (retropharyngeal lymph node dissection) is not yet reachable by the 3Dees approach due to the absence of ad hoc designed surgical instruments, and the poor ergonomics when using the mechanical holder for VITOM.

6.5 Conclusions

The exoscopic approach using VITOM for oropharyngeal procedures can be considered an excellent alternative to the operating microscope and robotic surgery, with its excellent performance in visual translation, depth of field, magnification, image contrast and color. Purchase cost is reduced as VITOM is about 10 times less expensive than a Da Vinci robotic platform. The system is not bulky and the operator can use all conventional surgical instruments. Furthermore, when combined with HD video endoscopy, the system provides excellent visualization via the monitor, and if available, a 3D camera can also be used to enhance images. Thanks to this system, anatomic details are clearer, and fine vascularization and irregularities of the mucosa become perfectly visible. It provides ample working space and is extremely useful for training and educational purposes. This technique is extremely beneficial in the learning process, especially for residents, as it provides the same visual experience for all operators, and tutors can pilot the learners' surgical maneuvers.

The 3Dees approach can be added to the other established strategies for transoral resection of oropharyngeal squamous cell carcinoma and can also have immediate and straightforward application in non oncologic surgical procedures (tonsillectomy, lateral pharyngoplasty, etc.).

The exoscopic platform has been improved thanks to the development of 10 mm diameter 3D optics (0 −30 degrees) useful to treat those cancers in the tonsillar region toward the base of the tongue and vallecula.

Further research must be oriented to the development of an electromagnetic holder that makes the positioning of the exoscope quick, precise, and responsive.

References

1. Elrefaey S, Massaro MA, Chiocca S, et al. HPV in oropharyngeal cancer: the basics to know in clinical practice. *Acta Otorhinolaryngol Ital*. 2014;34(5):299−309.
2. Sturgis EM, Ang KK. The epidemic of HPV-associated oropharyngeal cancer is here: is it time to change our treatment paradigms? *J Natl Compr Canc Netw*. 2011;9(6):665−673.
3. van Monsjou HS, van Velthuysen ML, van den Brekel MW, et al. Oropharyngeal squamous cell carcinoma: a unique disease on the rise? *Oral Oncol*. 2010;46(11):780−785.

4. Robinson KL, Macfarlane GJ. Oropharyngeal cancer incidence and mortality in Scotland: are rates still increasing? *Oral Oncol.* 2003;39(1):31−36.
5. Stransky N, Egloff AM, Tward AD, et al. The mutational landscape of head and neck squamous cell carcinoma. *Science.* 2011;333(6046):1157−1160.
6. McKiernan J, Thom B. CE: human papillomavirus-related oropharyngeal cancer: a review of nursing considerations. *Am J Nurs.* 2016;116(8):34−43.
7. Huet P. L'électro-coagulation dans les épithéliomas de l'amygdale palatine. *Ann Otolaryngol.* 1951;68:433−442.
8. Ryu CH, Ryu J, Cho KH, et al. Human papillomavirus-related cell cycle markers can predict survival outcomes following a transoral lateral oropharyngectomy for tonsillar squamous cell carcinoma. *J Surg Oncol.* 2014;110(4):393−399.
9. Laccourreye O, Hans S, Ménard M, et al. Transoral lateral oropharyngectomy for squamous cell carcinoma of the tonsillar region: II. An analysis of the incidence, related variables, and consequences of local recurrence. *Arch Otolaryngol Head Neck Surg.* 2005;131(7):592−599.
10. Laccourreye O, Malinvaud D, Holostenco V, et al. Value and limits of non-robotic transoral oropharyngectomy for local control of T1-2 invasive squamous cell carcinoma of the tonsillar fossa. *Eur Ann Otorhinolaryngol Head Neck Dis.* 2015;132(3):141−146.
11. Steiner W, Fierek O, Ambrosch P, Hommerich CP, Kron N. Transoral laser microsurgery for squamous cell carcinoma of the base of the tongue. *Arch Otolaryngol Head Neck Surg.* 2003;129(1):36−43.
12. Hockstein NG, Weinstein GS, O'Malley Jr BW. Maintenance of hemostasis in transoral robotic surgery. *ORL J Otorhinolaryngol Relat Spec.* 2005;67(4):220−224.
13. Hockstein NG, Nolan JP, O'Malley Jr BW, et al. Robotic microlaryngeal surgery: a technical feasibility study using the daVinci surgical robot and an airway mannequin. *Laryngoscope.* 2005;115(5):780−785.
14. O'Malley Jr BW, Weinstein GS, Snyder W, et al. Transoral robotic surgery (TORS) for base of tongue neoplasms. *Laryngoscope.* 2006;116(8):1465−1472.
15. Weinstein GS, O'Malley Jr BW, Snyder W, et al. Transoral robotic surgery: radical tonsillectomy. *Arch Otolaryngol Head Neck Surg.* 2007;133(12):1220−1226.
16. Moore EJ, Hinni ML. Critical review: transoral laser microsurgery and robotic-assisted surgery for oropharynx cancer including human papillomavirus-related cancer. *Int J Radiat Oncol Biol Phys.* 2013;85(5):1163−1167.
17. Genden EM, Desai S, Sung CK. Transoral robotic surgery for the management of head and neck cancer: a preliminary experience. *Head Neck.* 2009;31(3):283−289, 20.
18. Iseli TA, Kulbersh BD, Iseli CE, et al. Functional outcomes after transoral robotic surgery for head and neck cancer. *Otolaryngol Head Neck Surg.* 2009;141(2):166−171.
19. Moore EJ, Olsen KD, Kasperbauer JL. Transoral robotic surgery for oropharyngeal squamous cell carcinoma: a prospective study of feasibility and functional outcomes. *Laryngoscope.* 2009;119(11):2156−2164.
20. Boudreaux BA, Rosenthal EL, Magnuson JS, et al. Robot-assisted surgery for upper aerodigestive tract neoplasms. *Arch Otolaryngol Head Neck Surg.* 2009;135(4):397−401.
21. Weinstein GS, O'Malley Jr BW, Magnuson JS, et al. Transoral robotic surgery: a multicenter study to assess feasibility, safety, and surgical margins. *Laryngoscope.* 2012;122(8):1701−1707.
22. Moore EJ, Olsen SM, Laborde RR, et al. Long-term functional and oncologic results of transoral robotic surgery for oropharyngeal squamous cell carcinoma. *Mayo Clin Proc.* 2012;87(3):219−225.

23. Kim WS, Byeon HK, Park YM, et al. Therapeutic robot-assisted neck dissection via a retroauricular or modified facelift approach in head and neck cancer: a comparative study with conventional transcervical neck dissection. *Head Neck.* February 2015;37(2): 249–254.
24. Byeon HK, Holsinger FC, Kim DH, et al. Feasibility of robot-assisted neck dissection followed by transoral robotic surgery. *Br J Oral Maxillofac Surg.* January 2015;53(1): 68–73.
25. Goh HK, Ng YH, Teo DT. Minimally invasive surgery for head and neck cancer. *Lancet Oncol.* March 2010;11(3):281–286.
26. Blanco RG, Boahene K. Robotic-assisted skull base surgery: preclinical study. *J Laparoendosc Adv Surg Tech A.* 2013;23(9):776–782.
27. Krishnan KG, Scholler K, Uhl E. Application of a compact high-definition exoscope for illumination and magnification in high-precision surgical procedures. *World Neurosurg.* 2017;97:652–660.
28. Rossini Z, Cardia A, Milani D, Lasio GB, Fornari M, D'Angelo V. VITOM3D: preliminary experience in cranial surgery. *World Neurosurg.* 2017;107:663–668.
29. Ricciardi L, Chaichana KL, Cardia A, et al. The exoscope in neurosurgery: an innovative "point of view". A systematic review of the technical, surgical, and educational aspects. *World Neurosurg.* 2019;124:136–144.
30. Frykman PK, Duel BP, Gangi A, et al. Evaluation of a video telescopic operating microscope (VITOM) for pediatric surgery and urology: a preliminary report. *J Laparoendosc Adv Surg Tech A.* 2013;23(7):639–643.
31. Carlucci C, Fasanella L, Ricci Maccarini A. Exolaryngoscopy: a new technique for laryngeal surgery. *Acta Otorhinolaryngol Ital.* 2012;32(5):326–328.
32. Tasca I, Ceroni Compadretti G, Romano C. High-definition video telescopic rhinoplasty. *Acta Otorhinolaryngol Ital.* 2016;36(6):496–498.
33. Crosetti E, Arrigoni G, Manca A, Caracciolo A, Bertotto I, Succo G. 3D exoscopic surgery (3Des) for transoral oropharyngectomy. *Front Oncol.* January 31, 2020;10:16.

CHAPTER

7 Exoscope-assisted middle ear surgery

Giovanni Colombo, MD [1,2], Matteo Di Bari, MD [1,2], Fabio Ferreli, MD [1,2]
[1]*Department of Biomedical Sciences, Humanitas University, Pieve Emanuele, Milan, Italy;*
[2]*Otorhinolaryngology Unit, IRCCS Humanitas Clinical and Research Center, Rozzano, Milan, Italy*

7.1 Historical background

In ear surgery, optical magnification and stereopsis are essential in identifying anatomical structures and performing surgical procedures safely and successfully.

The need for stereopsis and the importance of three-dimensional perception of the complex anatomy of the ear during surgery was firstly recognized 150 years ago, in 1869, by the Italian Emilio De Rossi.[1] This concept was brought to clinical practice approximately 50 years later when Carl Olof Nylen adapted the first dissecting microscope for use in otology, recognizing the need for magnification.[2] The operating microscope has been the optical system indissolubly linked to ear surgery since 1921.[3] Several improvements through the years led to the actual binocular high-definition microscope, which is a standard equipment in any ENT operating room worldwide.

Although the concepts of ear surgery and the classification of tympanoplasty have been defined, Ohnsorge at the Würzburg ENT clinic (1977) was the first to describe the intraoperative use of a new tool in ear surgery: the endoscope. From the early 1990s, endoscopic ear surgery has gained increasing popularity "to look around the corner," allowing new anatomical insight and perspectives of the middle ear structures. From that time, the endoscope was used to perform ear surgery exclusively or in adjunct to the surgical microscope.[4–7]

In the last decade, the implementation of modern video technology as the 4K high-definition and three-dimensional video has allowed to gain further importance to endoscope-guided surgery. Moreover, this technological advance introduced a new surgical tool in the field of surgical technology: the exoscope. The exoscope has been largely used in the field of neurosurgery in the recent years. However, even if exoscope-assisted ear surgery was recently introduced, it will take time to see the full expression of its potential.[8–12]

7.2 Principles

The operating microscope is an optical system of lenses that guarantee to the surgeon a stereoscopic sharp vision of the minute structures of the middle ear with

Exoscope-Assisted Surgery in Otorhinolaryngology. https://doi.org/10.1016/B978-0-323-83168-0.00008-2

natural colors. The magnification obtained with the microscope reduces the surgical field wideness with a deterioration of panoramic view while preserving the image quality. The microscope field of view is reduced when the magnification rise, in a cone-shaped fashion, as it is shown in Fig. 7.1A and D in endoauricular and postauricular approaches, respectively.

The exoscope is an extracorporeal video telescope, composed of an optical stereoscopic system made with a rigid rod lens with high-resolution image sensors, and an integrated illumination with optical fibers. It is suspended above the surgical field while it produces high-quality full-HD three-dimensional images. These images are visualized on a large-format HD 4K resolution flat screen by the surgeon and the other operating room staff wearing 3D glasses. It can provide good image quality, lighting, and focal and field depth. The magnification is at first optical, while it becomes digital as it increases (2–16×). This allows for higher preservation of field wideness while increasing magnification (parallelepiped shape), thanks also to the "intraoperative navigation" within the surgical field allowed by the IMAGE1 PILOT (Fig. 7.1B and E).

The rigid ear endoscopes are the tubular fiber-optical instrument with different angulation of view (scopes 0 degrees, 30 degrees, 45 degrees, 70 degrees, etc.) that are introduced deep in the surgical cavity to explore the middle ear with a close high-detailed view that has the shape of an inverted angled cone (Fig. 7.1C and F).

The microscope allows for the best high magnification rendering. However, there is a reduction of the field wideness increasing the magnification, and only those structures that can be placed directly in the line of the light cone can be visualized. Surgery can be performed through all surgical corridors with appropriate depth perception and image quality with the right microscope adjustments. This is the reason why it is the gold standard in all ear surgical procedures nowadays.

The exoscope can provide an extremely detailed high-quality image, preserving a panoramic view of the surgical field during the procedures. The images are digitally elaborated and thus less natural than an operative microscope, especially at high magnification due to the current limits of digital zoom (Fig. 7.2). If high magnification is needed, the gain rises resulting in image definition, contrast, and brightness that are inferior compared to the microscope optical magnification. The need for digital magnification can be minimized by moving the exoscope 3D camera as close as possible to the surgical field.

Overall, the exoscope compared to the operating microscope has the advantages of lightness, maneuverability, and compactness. It can be easily rotated and moved in any direction using one hand with the chance of achieving even narrow view angles. On the other hand, the exoscope needs a large surgical corridor to guarantee a good performance; otherwise, the use of a microscope should be preferred. That was the reason that guided us to select only postauricular approaches in exoscope-assisted ear surgery.[13]

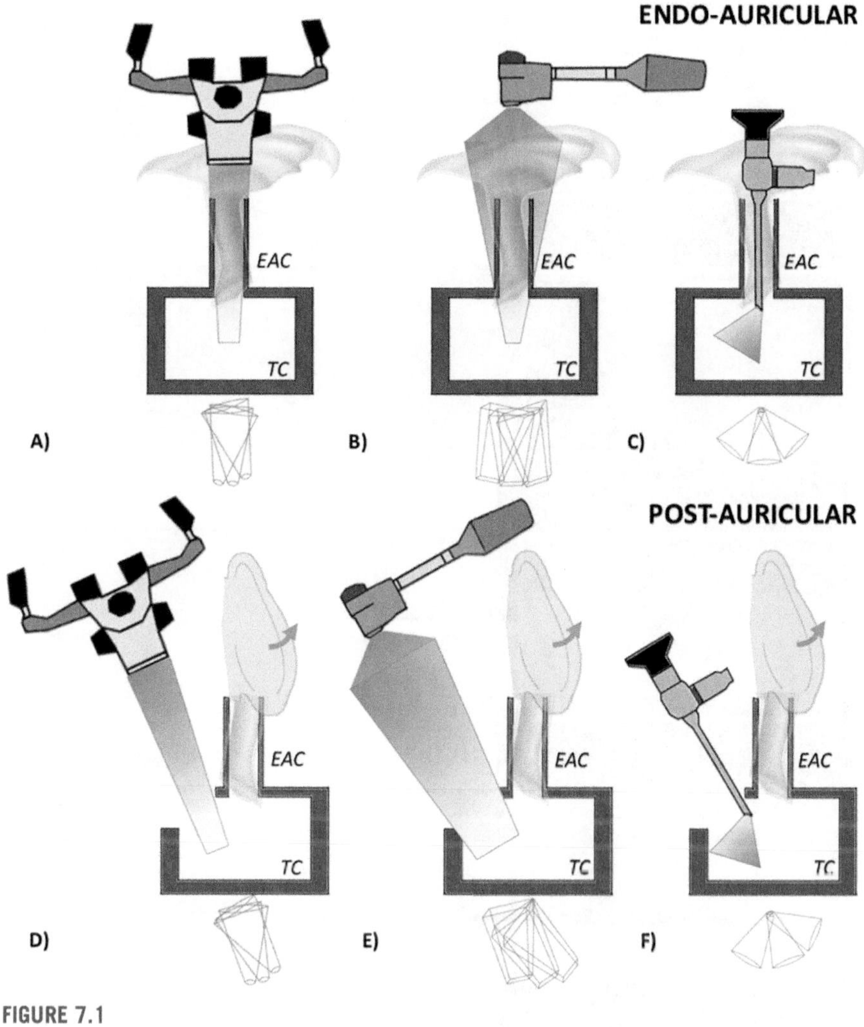

FIGURE 7.1

Endoauricular. Comparison of *endoauricular* field of view of the different magnification tools in ear surgery. (A) Microscope cone-shaped field of view. (B) Exoscope parallelepipedal field of view. (C) Endoscope inverted-cone field of view. The exoscope and the microscope determine the same wideness of the surgical field. Postauricular. Comparison of *postauricular* field of view of the different magnification tools in ear surgery. (D) Microscope cone-shaped field of view. (E) Exoscope parallelepipedal field of view. (F) Endoscope inverted-cone field of view. The exoscope allows for a more panoramic view in the postauricular approach when compared to other tools. *EAC*, external auditory canal; *TC*, tympanic cavity.

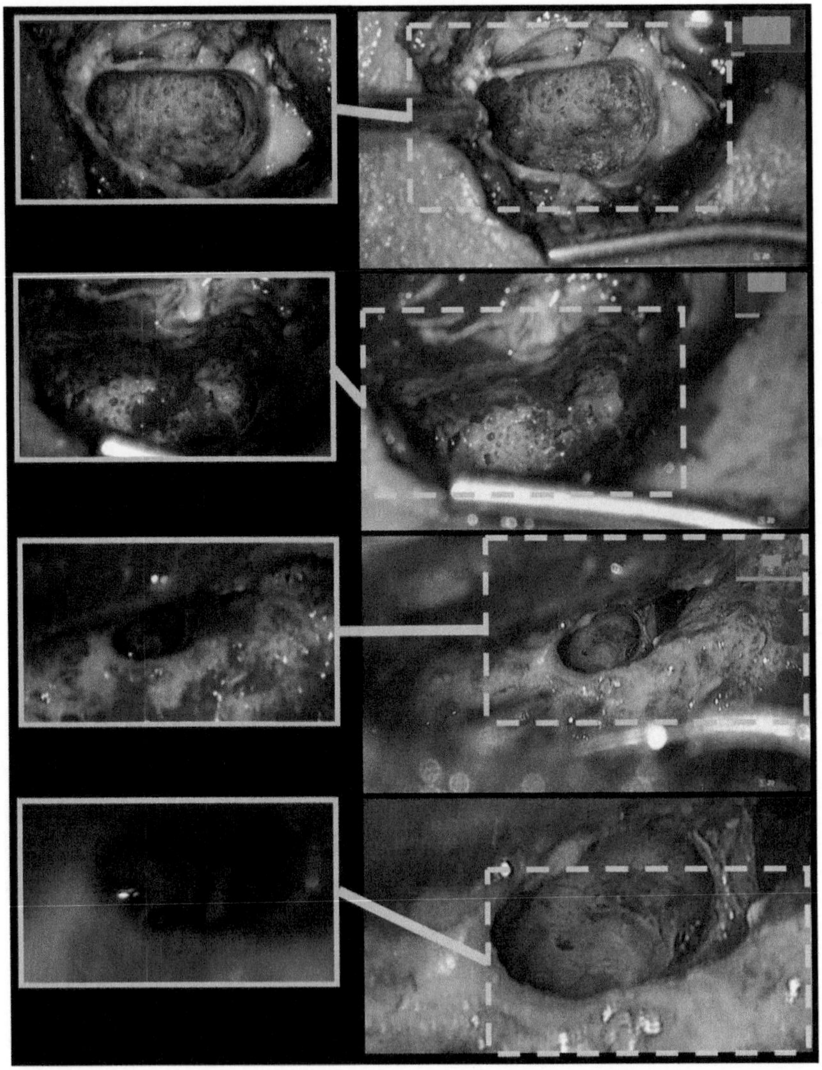

FIGURE 7.2

Step-by-step comparison of cochlear implant surgery in a left ear of a single patient. On the right column, surgical field as seen with exoscope (3D converted in 2D). On the left column, surgical field as seen with operating microscope. When the magnification increases, from top to bottom, the exoscope preserves a more panoramic view, but it has an inferior image quality when compared to the operating microscope. In the last row, the round window is well recognizable with both tools.

Image adapted from Colombo G, Ferreli F, Di Bari M, et al, Introducing the high-definition 3D exoscope in ear surgery: preliminary analysis of advantages and limits compared with operative microscope. Eur Arch Oto-Rhino-Laryngol *2020 (in press).*

An appropriate analogy can be made with smartphone technology versus professional camera. The combined use of optical and digital zoom is a technology in continuous improvement, with increased usage of the smartphone also in the professional photography and videomaking fields. The same is valid for the exoscope. Its technology can potentially have an exponential development in terms of image quality in all settings and magnification degrees, and this is the reason why it is a future-oriented tool.

The endoscope has different characteristics with respect to the other two tools. It allows to go through even narrower surgical corridors and to "look around corners," but it needs the use of one hand and it can determine the loss of depth perception and stereopsis. For these peculiar features, even if some surgeons use this tool as a stand-alone in their surgery, in our experience it is complementary to the others.[14] The highest versatility is ensured in combined exoscope–endoscope surgery, in which the use of the same video column and monitor allows a rapid and effective shift between these two tools, changing just the monitor source setting and the light source. The exoscope is a really intuitive system, and surgeons experienced in endoscopic surgery are more facilitate, given that surgeon and monitor positions are the same.

7.3 Indications and contraindications

The best suitable surgeries for exoscopic usage are postauricular approaches with mastoidectomy. These approaches enhance the qualities of this visualization and magnification instrument, providing a wide field for the detailed and panoramic view of the exoscope.

Endoauricular approaches are not yet suitable for exoscope-assisted surgery, due to both the narrow corridor and the need for a stereoscopic sharp vision of the middle ear minute structures with natural colors.

7.4 Operating room set-up

The operating room layout (Fig. 7.3A) starts from the necessity to have sufficient working space for the surgeon and the scrub nurse at the head of the patient. It has to ensure maximum efficiency and easy access to all resources, especially in case of adverse events during surgery.

The patient lies supine on an electrically operated surgical table, with the head rotated contralaterally with respect to the surgical side. The angle between head and shoulders has to be more than 90 degrees to allow for adequate working space. The patient's head has to be as close as possible to the surgeon and to the superior edge of the table. The patient should be maintained in the final desired position. The head rotation needed during surgery is achieved with the rotation of the operating room (OR) table, controlled by the OR nurse with a remote control positioned at the feet of the table.

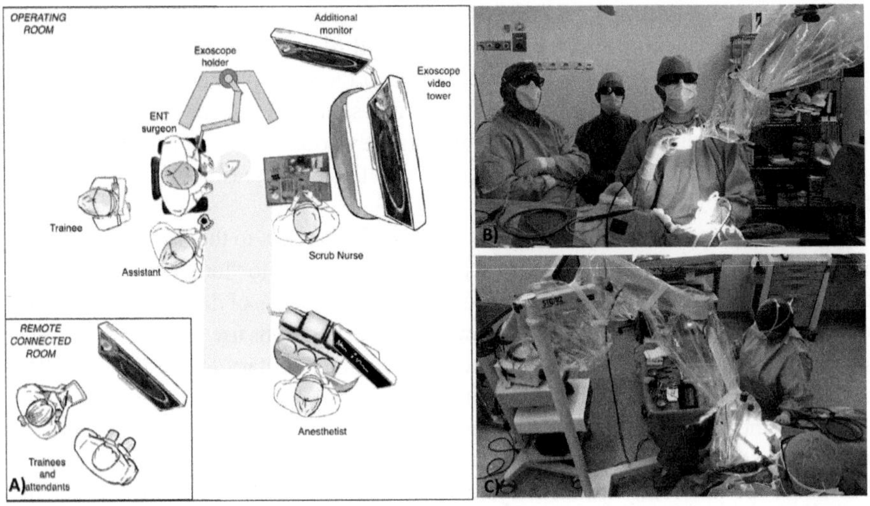

FIGURE 7.3

(A) Operating room layout. (B) Surgeon position. The camera can be easily adjusted and tilted with one hand. (C) Exoscope position from the top. The "S" shape allows for easy all-directions movements of the exoscope camera for the surgeon.

Image adapted from Colombo G, Ferreli F, Di Bari M, et al, Introducing the High-definition 3D exoscope in ear surgery: preliminary analysis of advantages and limits compared with operative microscope. Eur Arch Oto-Rhino-Laryngol *2020 (in press).*

The anesthetist, the anesthesia nurse, and all the anesthesia equipment are settled at the table feet, as in all head and neck surgeries. The endotracheal tube is secured to the mouth edge and to the patient's chest, while it is directed to the table feet, as well as the intravenous and other lines.

The surgeon sits in front of the surgical side at the table head. Stools can be adjusted or even removed in relation to the type of procedure and the surgeon's habit. The head is in a slight hyperextension toward the monitor, maintaining a natural posture (Fig. 7.3B). The surgeon needs to familiarize with this new position, even if it is similar to the position maintained during endoscopic procedures.

The scrub nurse stands on the other side of the surgical table, toward the table feet to not obstruct the surgeon's view of the monitor. The Mayo stand can be otherwise placed in front of the surgeon.

The surgeon and all the operating room staff should wear 3D glasses to be involved in the surgery.

The 3D exoscope is placed at the patient's head laterally to the surgeon, differently compared to the operating microscope standard position.[15] The camera is placed at the level of the surgeon's chest, avoiding hindering arms movements (see also exoscope positioning later).

The IMAGE1 PILOT system can be placed on the right or left in relation to the surgeon's preference, to easily maneuver it by himself or by the assistant, that usually stands on the first surgeon's side. The use of IMAGE1 PILOT by the assistant can increase the attention and the involvement in the surgery.

The video column with the 3D 4k monitor has to be positioned on the opposite side of the surgeon at the top of the surgical bed as shown in Figure 3. Supplementary 2D or 3D screens can be placed in different positions to allow the scrub nurse and assistants to have a good view.

In this operating room set-up, different working areas can be obtained with a proper space for the main surgeon, scrub nurse, assistant, and anesthetist. Observers can have a proper place behind the surgeon or at the feet of the table without interfering with the surgical act. Moreover, they share the same monitor and view of the main surgeon, achieving a 360-degrees experience in surgery. Additional monitors can expand even more the possibility of sharing, such as in the context of courses and live surgery sessions. This technology is also suitable to manage remote connections with rooms and lecture halls in the same hospital or in other institutions, with an adjunct of a speaker and microphone system to communicate with the surgeon. In fact, the exoscope can allow the same view and same field depth perception. A shared vision is crucial, especially in a teaching hospital with residency and fellowship programs, but also in every setting to enhance team collaboration and involvement in the surgery.

Another advantage in this operating room setting is that the set-up time and exoscope draping are comparable to that of the operating microscope.[13]

7.5 Exoscope positioning

The position of the holding system is different with respect to the operating microscope. In fact, the best position is on the same side of the surgeon to maximize the flexible use of the holding system arms. The arms have to be adjusted in an "S" shape position to maintain the second cantilever arm and the smaller "L" that holds the camera properly oriented over the surgical table, as seen in Fig. 7.3C.

Given this set-up, all movements of the smaller "L" are allowed, especially rotation on the axial plane ($\pm$90 degrees), and the different inclination needed during surgery. A handle at the distal extremity allows the 3D camera rotation to obtain a proper horizontal alignment during surgery. The buttons on the 3D camera could be easily reached with this positioning. Based on our experience, the best camera position is horizontal in front of the surgeon sternum, with the minimum focal distance (approximately 20 cm) to obtain the best image quality with the lower magnification. The camera should not be placed too close to the surgical field to not impair the surgeon's hands movement.

Once the exoscope is settled in the desired position, then it should be partially blocked to allow for controlled adjustments and avoid freely movements. In particular, after the ceiling, the holding system allows for an easy and precise individual final adjustment of the exoscope with its flexible layout, even with a single hand.

7.6 Surgical technique: postauricular approach

Postauricular approach is the best suitable for exoscopic surgery. The choice of this approach mirrors the proper technical features of the exoscope (see Section 7.2).

After the induction of general anesthesia and before draping, the postauricular area is injected with 2% lidocaine with 1:100,000 epinephrine. The exoscope can be used for all operative steps, from incision to skin closure. The head is positioned as close as possible to the surgical field to take full advantage of the optical zoom. The parallelepipedal vision allows to include in the surgical field view all the length of postauricular sulcus and even the entire pinna. The focus is adjusted through the IMAGE1 PILOT, and a precise skin incision is made along the hairline, approximately 5 mm behind the postauricular sulcus.

The Clara plus Chroma video setting can be useful in the following steps, because it can allow an enhanced view of the muscle and fascia due to a better visualization of red structures, and hemostasis can be achieved faster (Fig. 7.4). The video settings can be easily switched from the IMAGE1 PILOT buttons.

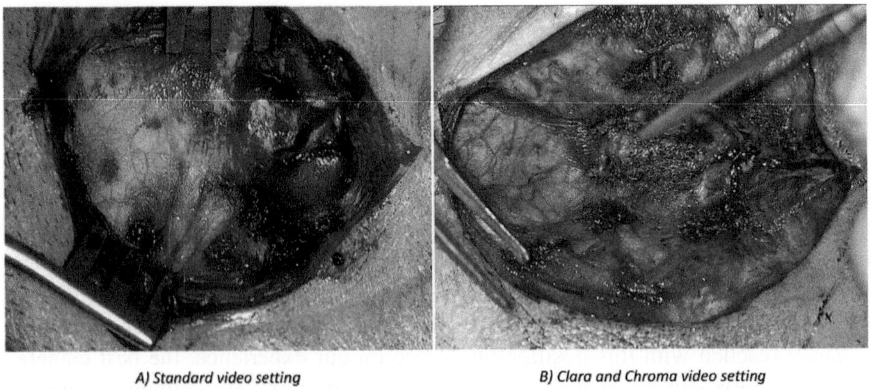

FIGURE 7.4

Comparison between fibromuscular layer image rendering between (A) Standard video setting and (B) Clara plus Chroma video setting. Right ear, different patients.

After a lateral sliding of the exoscope camera on the horizontal axis, the temporalis muscle fascia is harvested through an incision above the linea temporalis leaving about 1 cm of intact fascia to facilitate the closure of the postauricular incision. The fascia is elevated from the underlying temporalis muscle using the proper plane to minimize bleeding. The superior incision is made using curved scissors. On a block near the surgical field, extra tissue on the fascia can be trimmed and cut to the desired shape under exoscopic vision.

An inferiorly pedicled retroauricular periosteal flap is raised with an incision of musculoperiosteal tissue overlying the mastoid cortex. The flap does not have to include the underlying temporalis muscle to avoid necrosis (anteriorly vascularization by the deep temporalis arteries). The muscle is well defined without any particular magnification. The periosteal flap is elevated from the bone with a good exposition of the mastoid tip inferiorly, zygomatic line superiorly, and Henle's spine anteriorly. The cribriform area can also be identified.

At this step, a reduced brightness is needed to better visualize the bone. It can be useful to switch from Clara and Chroma to Standard video setting and to slightly increase the operative distance. These adjustments are crucial, especially in the case of the ivory mastoid.[13] An ivory mastoid is the sclerosis and loss of aeration of the mastoid air cells. The bone is compact and very bright with an unpleasant light reflex in the exoscope image.

When the mastoid is well exposed and a proper bone visualization is achieved, the mastoidectomy can start. We drill the mastoid within the triangle bounded superiorly by the tegmen mastoid, posteriorly by the sigmoid sinus, and anteriorly by the posterior wall of the ear canal to proceed with an intact canal mastoidectomy. During mastoidectomy it has to be maintained a correct and stable inclination of the 3D camera similarly to the operative microscope, especially approaching the vertical portion of the facial nerve canal. A proper angle is needed to correctly identify the facial nerve and avoid any damage. The high maneuvrability of the camera can lead to approach this step with an incorrect inclination, expecially at the beginning of the learning curve of exoscopic surgery.[13] The exoscope has to be settled in a position in which the resulting image is perpendicular to the posterior wall of the ear canal during these steps. At this point, a posterior tympanotomy can be performed if the aim is to approach the tympanic cavity (Fig. 7.5A).

The size and maneuverability of the exoscope camera and its wide angle of rotation (higher than the microscope) can allow a wider view of the middle ear microstructures through posterior tympanotomy, as it has been shown before in Fig. 7.2. This can be particularly helpful in the cholesteatoma removal, and in the exposure of the round window membrane in cochlear implants, especially when it has a downward inclination[13] (Fig. 7.5B).

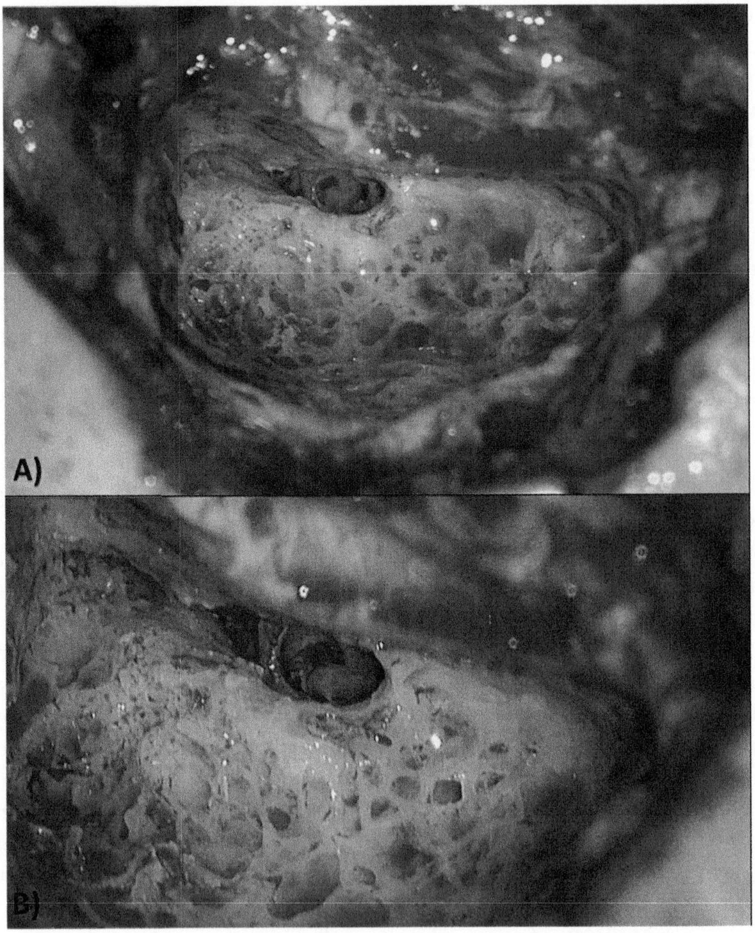

FIGURE 7.5

(A) Posterior tympanotomy. (B) Greater magnification showing round window exposition in cochlear implantation surgery. Right ear.

On the other hand, the higher magnification needed in this step determines a decrease of the image quality, when compared to the microscope. This unfavorable aspect due to the digital zoom is of less importance in canal wall-down mastoidectomy, because of the wide panoramic view achieved with the approach and maintained by the exoscope (Fig. 7.6).

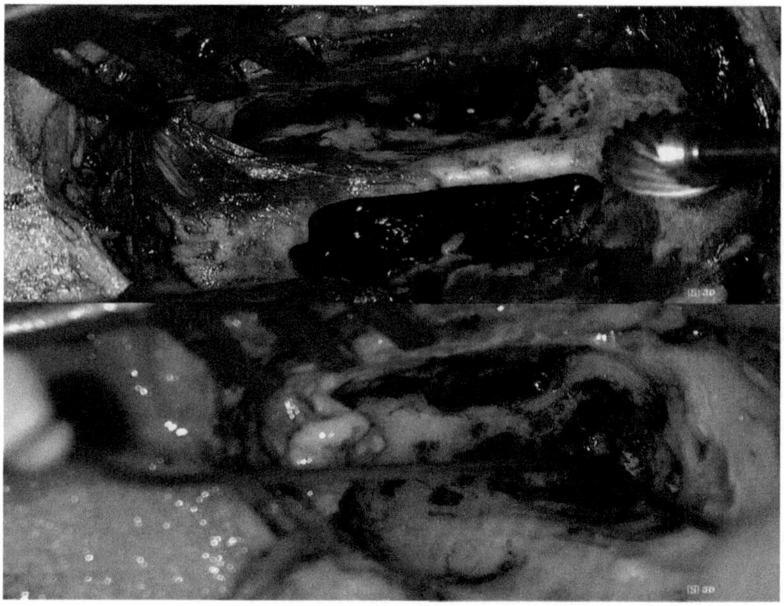

FIGURE 7.6

Comparison of canal wall-up and canal wall-down mastoidectomy exoscope view.

7.7 Conclusions

The exoscope is safe and efficient in treating diseases of the middle ear through post-auricular approaches, allowing for an easy involvement of the surgical team, trainee, and observers. On the other hand, exoscope-assisted middle ear surgery has still some limitations that can probably be overcome by the technology evolution. The wider variation of vision angle in exoscope surgery requires the definition of new anatomical point of views with specific training. It should be taken into account a lengthening of some procedure's steps during the early experience.

The exoscope is not yet a tool capable to substitute the operative microscope, but it represents an additional, innovative tool to be added to ear surgical equipment. The recent development of exoscopic robotic arms is just the first step in a process of technological evolution that is just begun.

References

1. De Rossi E. L'otoscopie binoculaire. *Monatsschr Ohrenheil.* 1869;3:170–172.
2. Dohlman G. Carl Olof Nylen and the birth of the otomicroscope and microsurgery. *Arch Otolaryngol.* 1969;90:813–817.
3. Mudry A. The history of the microscope for use in ear surgery. *Am J Otol.* 2000;21(6): 877–886.

4. Ohnsorge P. Intraoperative endoscopy of middle-ear and endoscopic diagnostic of middle-ear by a new endoscopic unit. *Arch Otorhinolaryngol*. 1977;216:511.
5. Thomassin JM, Korchia D, Doris JM. Endoscopic guided otosurgery in the prevention of residual cholesteatomas. *Laryngoscope*. 1993;103:939–943.
6. Tarabichi M. Endoscopic management of acquired cholesteatoma. *Am J Otol*. 1997; 18(5):544–549.
7. Preyer S. Endoscopic ear surgery - a complement to microscopic ear surgery. *HNO*. 2017; 65(Suppl 1):29–34.
8. Ricciardi L, Chaichana KL, Cardia A, et al. The exoscope in neurosurgery: an innovative "point of view". A systematic review of the technical, surgical and educational aspects. *World Neurosurg*. 2019. S1878-8750(19)30080-30084.
9. Rubini A, Di Gioia S, Marchioni D. 3D exoscopic surgery of lateral skull base. *Eur Arch Otorhinolaryngol*. 2020;277(3):687–694.
10. Smith S, Kozin ED, Kanumuri VV, et al. Initial experience with 3-dimensional exoscope-assisted transmastoid and lateral skull base surgery. *Otolaryngol Head Neck Surg*. 2019; 160(2):364–367.
11. Garneau JC, Laitman BM, Cosetti MK, Hadjipanayis C, Wanna G. The use of the exoscope in lateral skull base surgery: advantages and limitations. *Otol Neurotol*. 2019; 40(2):236–240.
12. Minoda R, Miwa T. Non-microscopic middle ear cholesteatoma surgery: a case report of a novel head-up approach. *Otol Neurotol*. 2019;40(6):777–781.
13. Colombo G, Ferreli F, Di Bari M, et al. Introducing the high-definition 3D exoscope in ear surgery: preliminary analysis of advantages and limits compared with operative microscope. *Eur Arch Otorhinolaryngol*. 2020 (in press).
14. Poletti AM, Solimeno LS, Cugini G, Miceli S, Colombo G. Microendoscopic surgery of middle ear and petrous bone: benefits analysis. *Ear Nose Throat J*. 2020. https://doi.org/10.1177/0145561320930017.
15. *Glasscock-Shambaugh. Surgery of the Ear*. 5th ed. 2003:268–271 (chapter 12).

CHAPTER

Exoscopic surgery of lateral skull base

8

Daniele Marchioni, MD, Nicola Bisi, MD, Gabriele Molteni, MD, PhD FEBORL-HNO, Alessia Rubini, MD

Department of Otolaryngology, Head and Neck Surgery, University of Verona, Verona, Italy

8.1 Introduction

Literature includes some studies about the use of an exoscope in neurosurgery, either as an exclusive instrument or in combination with the microscope.[1–3]

The use of the operative exoscope has recently been introduced in head and neck surgery, and there are only a few studies in the literature regarding this kind of exoscopic surgery. Lateral skull-base surgery is traditionally performed mainly using the operative microscope, in some cases with endoscopic assistance.

Some of the limitations of the operative microscope are its large frame and its fixed cumbersome design. It also forces the primary surgeon and his assistants to have fixed positions around the operative field with limited visual angles. Moreover, the operative microscope screens oblige the assistants to follow the surgical procedure with a two-dimensional view because only the surgeon has a stereoscopic vision.

Conversely, endoscopic surgery allows for an ergonomic position of the surgeon with a horizontal gaze and an angled vision "behind the corner."

Exoscopic surgery is a new surgical technique that has the purpose of using the exoscope to replace the microscope during surgical approaches, it requires the use of a classic two-handed surgery, as it happens in microscopic surgery, while looking at the monitor, where the exoscopic vision is shown.

Exoscopic surgery combines the features of an endoscopic surgical approach as the surgeon works looking at the monitor positioned in front of him/her and the microscopic surgical technique, because the surgeon works with two hands.

However, exoscopic surgery requires adequate training to learn the simultaneous coordination of the hands with the images appearing on the monitor. This technique needs previous training on endoscopic and microscopic surgery because the skills deriving from both techniques are necessary to perform surgery using the exoscope.

Exoscopes are produced by various companies and provide high-resolution imaging and two different kinds of view: two-dimensional (2D) or three-dimensional (3D).

In both the 2D and 3D exoscopes, the images are displayed on 4K high-definition monitors that can enhance anatomical details and make them more realistic.

Exoscope-Assisted Surgery in Otorhinolaryngology. https://doi.org/10.1016/B978-0-323-83168-0.00004-5

A 2D exoscope has a 2D vision that is not overcome by the movement of the instrument in the surgical field, as it happens in endoscopic surgery, so it is especially used for video recordings and teaching reasons. On the other hand, the use of a 3D exoscope has 3D vision and allows both residents and fellows to follow the surgical procedure in the same way as the first surgeon.

This chapter is based on our experience with the VITOM 3D exoscope (Karl Storz GmbH, Tuttlingen, Germany) system on lateral skull-base surgical management. We will here describe the use of exoscopic surgery in the surgical treatment of lateral skull-base lesions.

8.2 Exoscopic approaches to lateral skull base

A 3D exoscope can be used as an operative tool to perform surgical procedures in the lateral skull base, replacing the microscope in the majority of cases.

Like every operative tool, the exoscope presents both advantages and disadvantages.

8.2.1 Advantages

- The use of a 3D exoscope provides the surgeon and his assistants with the same three-dimensional images. It allows fellows and residents to follow the surgery in the same way as the first surgeon
- The anatomical structures are more realistic and the recognition and differentiation of the structures are better through a 3D exoscopic view than through a microscopic one.
- It has a small frame with a large depth of field, which reduces the need to refocus during periods of dissection.[2]
- Shifting from a microscopic to a macroscopic vision can be rapidly and easily done without moving the scope or completely losing microscopic vision.
- Its wide operative fields and focal distances are long enough to provide unobstructed operative corridors and enable the surgeon to have a considerable amount of mobility to work with the necessary tools.[4]
- It allows for an ergonomic position of the surgeon with a horizontal gaze throughout the surgical operation. The horizontal gaze may be also maintained throughout surgery using an operative microscope; however, the use of fixed optics limits head and neck movement causing discomfort to the surgeon.[1]

8.2.2 Disadvantages

- A high-intensity light can cause homogenization of the colors and the anatomical structures in the surgical field, so a proper regulation of the light is necessary.
- Lighting is low in the case of small surgical corridors, and pixelation can occur at high magnification in lateral skull base and mastoid surgery (e.g., in the case of posterior tympanotomy).[5]

- The depth perception using a 3D exoscopic visualization at the highest magnification is inferior to the one provided by a standard operative microscope.
- Minimal dizziness, little nausea, fatigue, or vertigo have been described in some studies using a 3D vision during surgery.[6]
- It provides a direct view of the surgical field, like the microscope while the endoscope allows visual control around corners.

In this complex area, both the microscope and the exoscope present the same difficult visualization of the hidden areas (medial to the tympanic and labyrinthine tracts of the facial nerve, medial to the vertical and horizontal segments of the internal carotid artery in the petrous bone). For this reason, it is often necessary to perform an endoscopic check of the surgical field with an angled endoscope at the end of the exoscopic or microscopic procedures to detect any potential residual pathology, which might be located in nonvisualized areas.

8.2.3 Exoscopic surgery of the lateral skull base: rationale

Lateral cranial base surgery often requires surgical skills, and a deep knowledge of the anatomy of the neck, the temporal bone, the petrous apex, and of the cerebellopontine angle (CPA). There are quite a few lateral skull-base pathologies; among them, the most frequent ones are acoustic neuromas, cholesterol granulomas, petrous bone cholesteatomas, temporal bone paragangliomas, facial nerve tumors, etc.

In most cases, the approaches to the lateral cranial base require the use of the operative microscope (translabyrinthine, transotic, transcochlear, middle cranial fossa, retrosigmoid approaches). Recently, exclusively endoscopic procedures have been introduced for few selected cases (transcanal transpromontorial approach for limited acoustic neuromas and transcanal suprageniculate approach for limited geniculate ganglion tumors or selected posttraumatic facial palsy for geniculate ganglion injury).

In many cases, because of the complex anatomy, in the same patient, the procedure requires the management of the neck and the temporal bone anatomy, performing a surgical step on the neck to isolate the major blood vessels and the extracranial tract of the nerves, at the exits from the foramina.

After the neck surgical step, it is possible to perform a wide microscopic demolition of the temporal bone to reach the pathological process. A typical example is Type A infratemporal fossa approach that is used for the management of lesions located at the level of the jugular foramen. During these procedures, the microscope is used only during the demolition of the temporal bone.

The introduction of exoscopic surgery has allowed the surgeon to replace the microscope during the demolition of the temporal bone and to perform the surgical steps in the neck with the same surgical instruments, with a more precise surgical outcome, through a 3D view.

Currently, a few studies are present in the literature, but a new promising surgical technique has been introduced for the management of the complex lateral skull-base pathological processes.

8.2.4 Operating room setup

VITOM 3D exoscope (Karl Storz GmbH, Tuttlingen, Germany) is used as an operative tool in lateral skull-base surgery. The system consists of a holding arm for VITOM 3D placed in front of the surgical field (at a distance of 20–50 cm). This is a full HD 3D, 16: 9 modular video system, stereoscopic optics with high-resolution image sensors (4K) and 8–30× magnification. The image is shown on a 3D monitor using the appropriate passive glasses.

The 3D 4K screen is placed in front of the surgeon allowing a direct view during surgery. The surgeon and the assistants wear 3D glasses or clip-on glasses for those wearing corrective glasses (Figs. 8.1 and 8.2).

There is a control unit (IMAGE PILOT), to either regulate the focus or to enlarge or shift the field of view. The latter is located next to the surgeon and kept in place by another holding arm. An assistant or the surgeon usually handles the control unit. If the assistant handles the control unit, the surgeon can focus only on the surgical procedure.

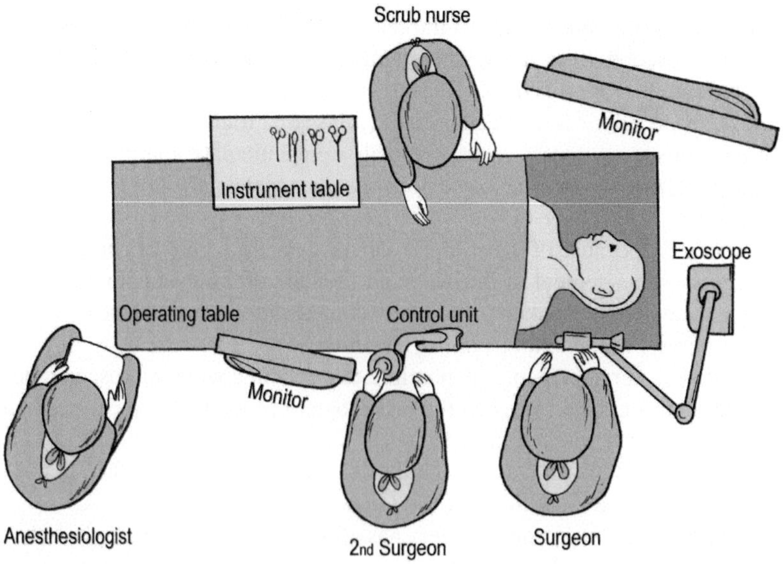

FIGURE 8.1

Diagram of the operating room setup showing the position of the exoscope, the control unit, and the video monitors in relation to the patient, the surgeons, the scrub nurse, and the anesthesiologist.

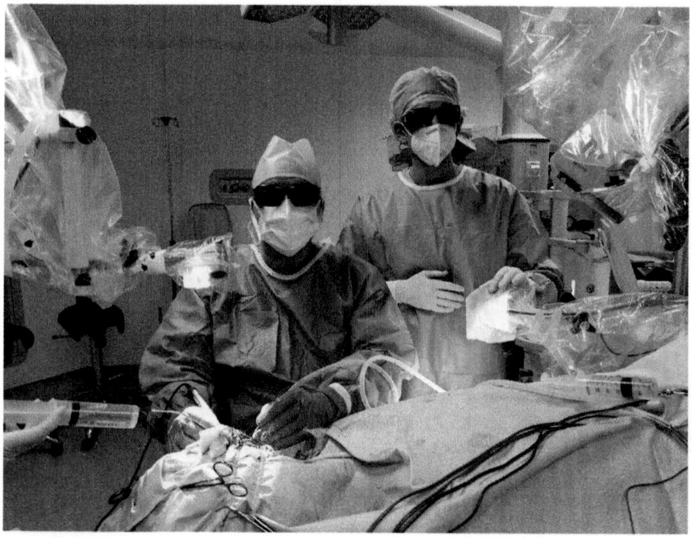

FIGURE 8.2

Operating room setup. The camera is attached to its holding arm and it is positioned on the surgeon's right side. The assistant stands on the left-hand side of the surgeon modifying both magnification and focus by using the control unit. Both the first surgeon and the assistant wear 3D glasses.

The surgical scrub nurse is on the opposite side of the operating table to the surgeon in front of a second 2D screen, while the anesthesiologist is at the foot of the operating bed (Fig. 8.3).

8.2.5 Surgical approaches to lateral skull base

The exoscope is best suited for approaches with a large surgical field, rather than for small surgical corridors, as in these cases it allows for an optimal replacement of the microscope.

Therefore, the surgeon works by looking at the high-definition monitor (4K) located in front of him/her (as it happens in endoscopic surgery) with a 3D view (as in microscopic surgery) working with two hands. Obviously, 3D exoscopic surgery requires adequate training.

From our experience, the surgical steps on soft tissue, bone tissue, and pathology dissection are easily feasible exclusively using the 3D exoscope instead of the traditional microscope in most of the procedures concerning the lateral skull base, as in the majority of these procedures a large surgical field without narrow corridors is required.

Transpetrous approaches can be divided as follows (Fig. 8.4):

- Posterior: retrosigmoid approach.

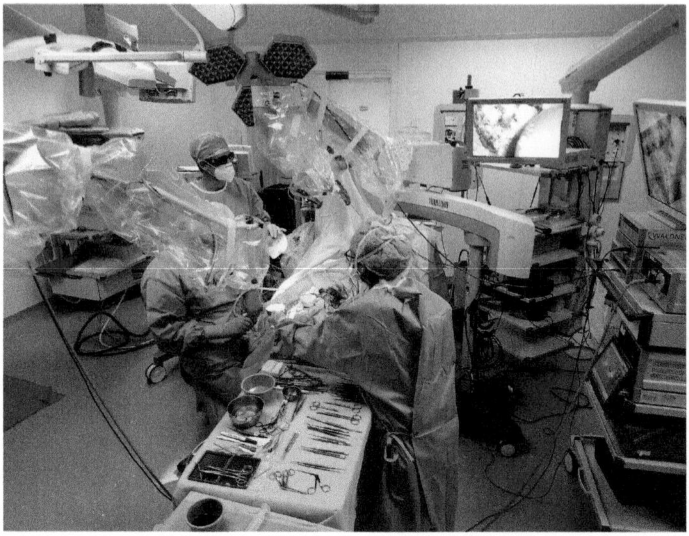

FIGURE 8.3

Operating room setup. The 3D monitor is in front of the surgeon and the assistant. The scrub nurse is on the opposite side of the surgeon following the surgery on an additional 2D video monitor.

- Lateral: retrolabyrinthine or presigmoid, translabyrinthine, transcochlear/transotic, transcanal transpromontorial, Fisch infratemporal fossa approach (type A, B, C, D approaches), subtotal petrosectomy.
- Anterior: middle cranial fossa approach, anterior petrosectomy.

Some of these approaches do not require a large surgical corridor, so exclusive exoscopic surgery is not as effective as the microscope for them (e.g., retrosigmoid approach), while for lateral and anterior transpetrous approaches the exoscope can replace the functions of the microscope. As it happens for microscopic surgery, exoscopic surgery, in some of transpetrous approaches, also needs an endoscopic assistance to explore the hidden areas and exclude any residual pathological process at the end of the procedure.

8.2.5.1 Type A, B, and C Fisch infratemporal fossa approaches

Type A Fisch infratemporal fossa (IFT) approach provides a good exposure of the jugular foramen area, and it is performed for benign or malignant tumor removal of this area (mostly benign tumors of the skull base, such as schwannomas or paragangliomas) (Figs. 8.5–8.13).

Type B Fisch IFT approach provides good exposure to benign lesions of the infratemporal fossa, clivus, petrous apex, while type C enables the surgeon to reach the pterygopalatine fossa, the parasellar region, and the nasopharynx. This group of procedures also includes a preauricular approach, type D IFT approach. This

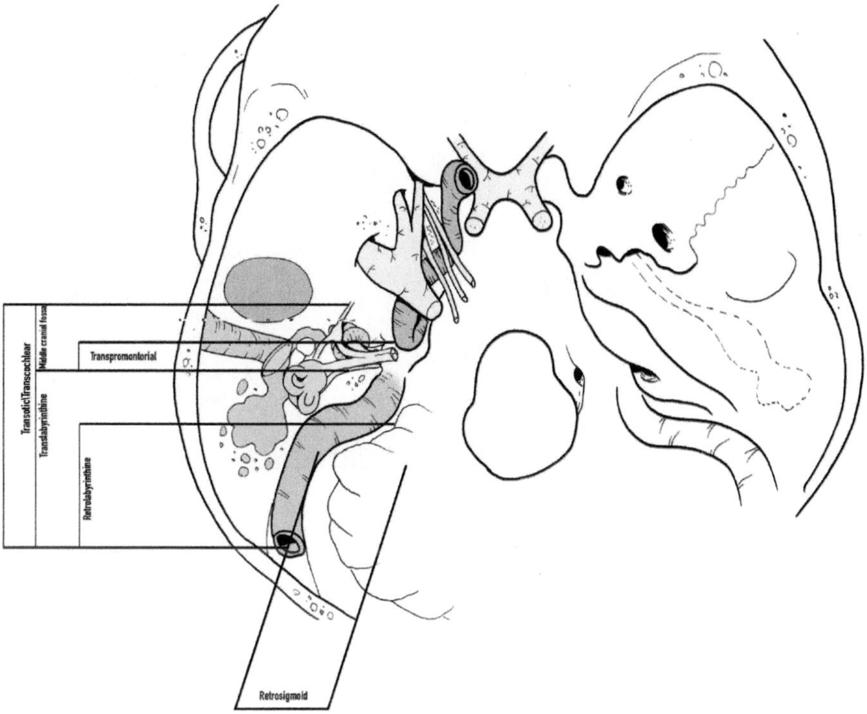

FIGURE 8.4

Drawing depicting the surgical corridors of the main transpetrous approaches to the lateral skull base and the anatomical landmarks encountered performing each of them. The posterior retrosigmoid approach, the lateral retrolabyrinthine, translabyrinthine, transotic and transcanal transpromontorial approaches, and the anterior middle cranial fossa approach are shown.

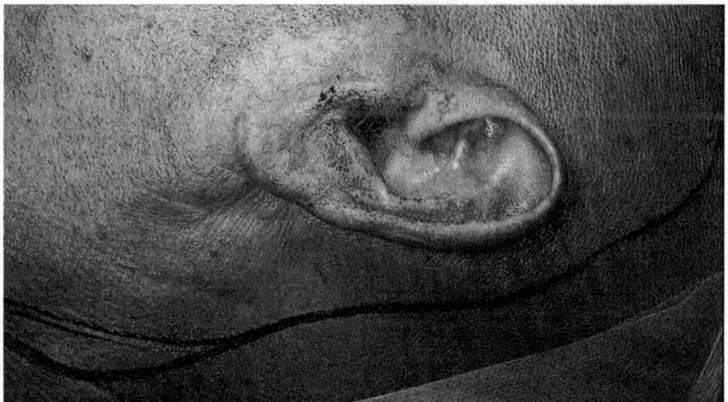

FIGURE 8.5

Type A Fisch infratemporal fossa approach, left side. The carnio temporo cervical skin incision is made as shown.

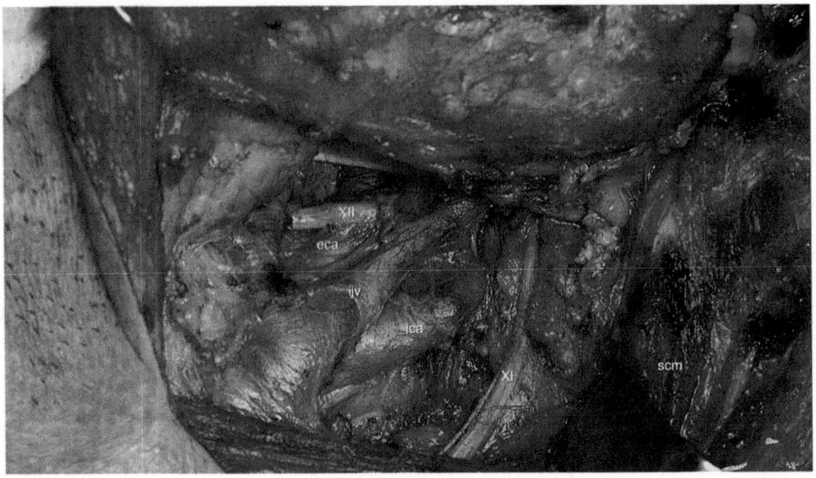

FIGURE 8.6

Type A Fisch infratemporal fossa approach, left side. The cervical step of this procedure is complete. The sternocleidomastoid muscle is posteriorly retracted, the internal jugular vein and the external and internal carotid arteries are identified in the neck along with the accessory spinal nerve and the hypoglossal nerve. *eca*, external carotid artery; *ica*, internal carotid artery; *ijv*, internal jugular vein; *scm*, sternocleidomastoid muscle; *XI*, XI cranial nerve; *XII*, XII cranial nerve.

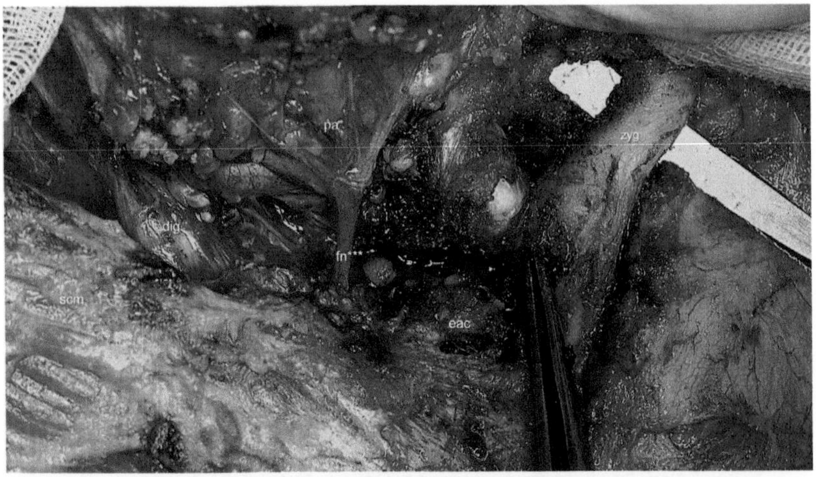

FIGURE 8.7

Type A Fisch infratemporal fossa approach, left side. This image shows the facial nerve trunk, as it exits the stylomastoid foramen at the same depth as one of the posterior bellies of the digastric muscle, and the start of the pes anserinus inside the parotid gland. The external auditory canal and the zygomatic process of the temporal bone are also displayed. *dig*, digastric muscle; *eac*, external auditory canal; *fn****, intraparotid facial nerve trunk; *pa*, parotid gland; *scm*, sternocleidomastoid muscle; *zyg*, zygomatic arch.

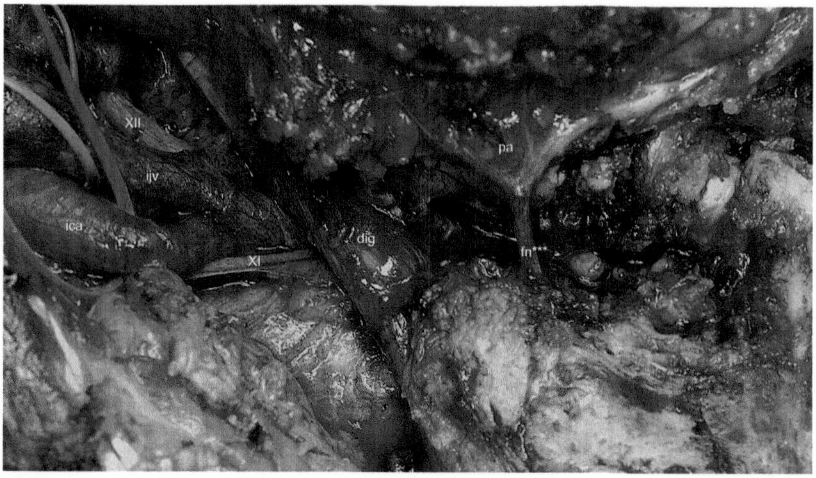

FIGURE 8.8

Type A Fisch infratemporal fossa approach, left side. A wide view of the dissection so far is shown, the internal jugular vein and the internal carotid artery are identified in the neck and marked with umbilical tapes, the hypoglossal nerve can be clearly seen, and the posterior belly of the digastric muscle, arising from the mastoid notch, and the facial nerve trunk are exhibited as well. *dig*, digastric muscle; *fn****, intraparotid facial nerve trunk; *ica*, internal carotid artery; *ijv*, internal jugular vein; *pa*, parotid gland; *XI*, XI cranial nerve; *XII*, XII cranial nerve.

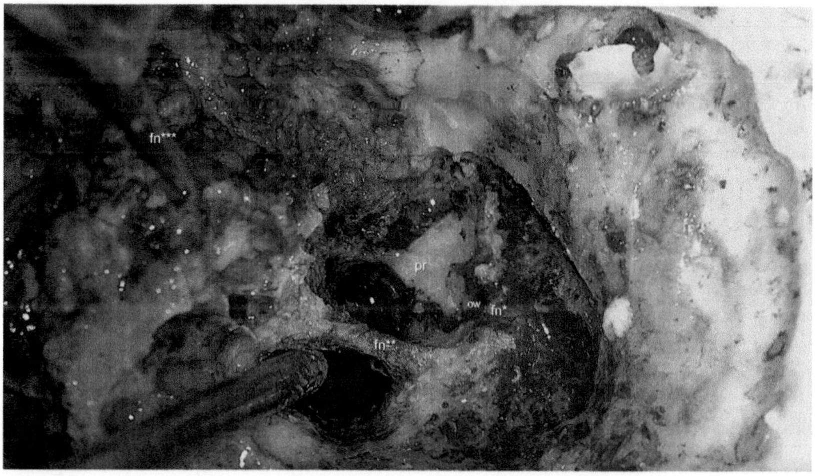

FIGURE 8.9

Type A Fisch infratemporal fossa approach, left side. A subtotal petrosectomy is performed, the promontory with its oval window is in view, and the mastoid segment of the facial nerve is left like a bridge inside the surgical field. This image shows how the infratemporal approach allows for a complete control of the facial nerve from its intraparotid segment, to its mastoid one, to the tympanic segment. *fn**, tympanic segment of facial nerve; *fn***, mastoid segment of facial nerve; *fn****, intraparotid facial nerve trunk; *pr*, promontory; *ow*, oval window.

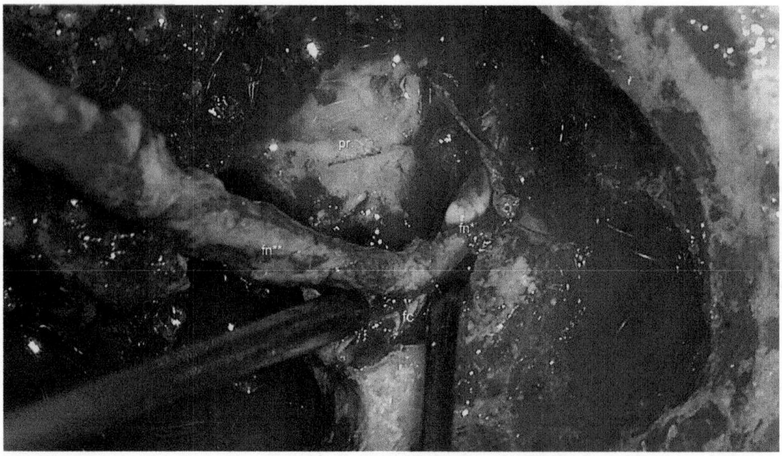

FIGURE 8.10

Type A Fisch infratemporal fossa approach, left side. The facial nerve has been skeletonized from the stylomastoid foramen to the geniculate ganglion. In this picture, the mastoid segment of the facial nerve is being carefully detached from the fallopian canal. *fn**, tympanic segment of facial nerve; *fn***, mastoid segment of facial nerve; *pr*, promontory.

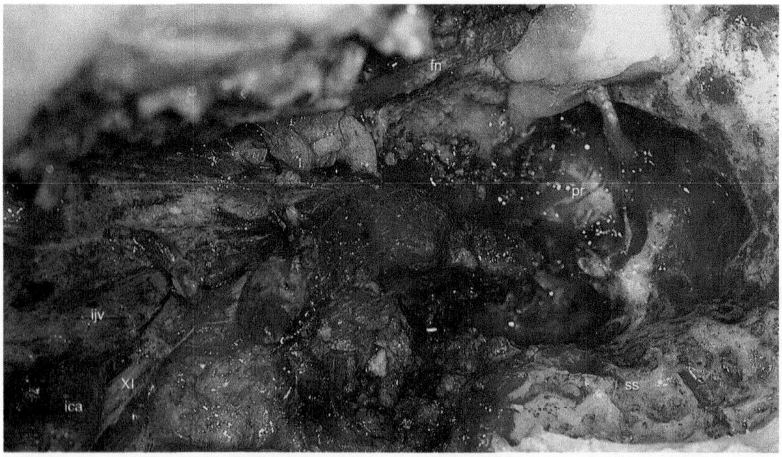

FIGURE 8.11

Type A Fisch infratemporal fossa approach, left side. Image showing the whole surgical field, the facial nerve has been anteriorly rerouted, and its bone canal has been drilled away to allow for proper control of the intrapetrous carotid artery. The sigmoid sinus can be seen as a blue hue in the inferior part of the surgical field. The neurovascular structures of the neck are visible as well. *fn*, rerouted facial nerve; *ica*, internal carotid artery; *ijv*, internal jugular vein; *pr*, promontory; *ss*, sigmoid sinus; *XI*, XI cranial nerve.

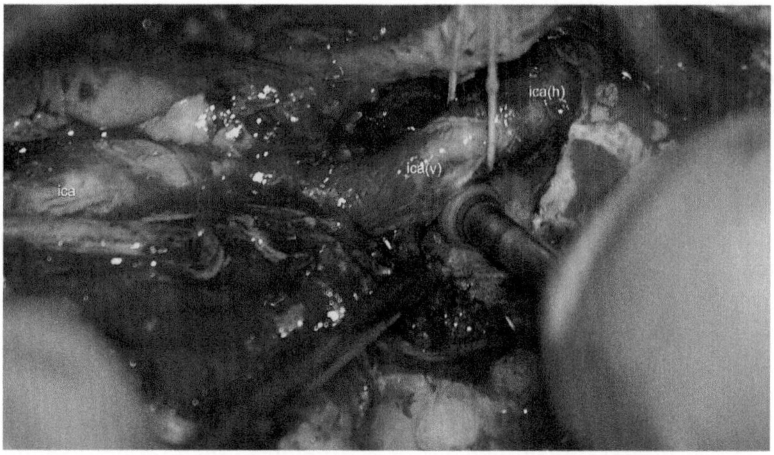

FIGURE 8.12

Type A Fisch infratemporal fossa approach, left side. The internal carotid artery is completely exposed from its cervical portion to part of its intrapetrous horizontal segment. This image shows the petrous apex and the clival region drilling medial to the vertical segment of the ICA to ensure a radical removal of the lesion. *ica*, internal carotid artery; *ica(h)*, horizontal tract of intrapetrous carotid artery; *ica(v)*, vertical tract of intrapetrous carotid artery.

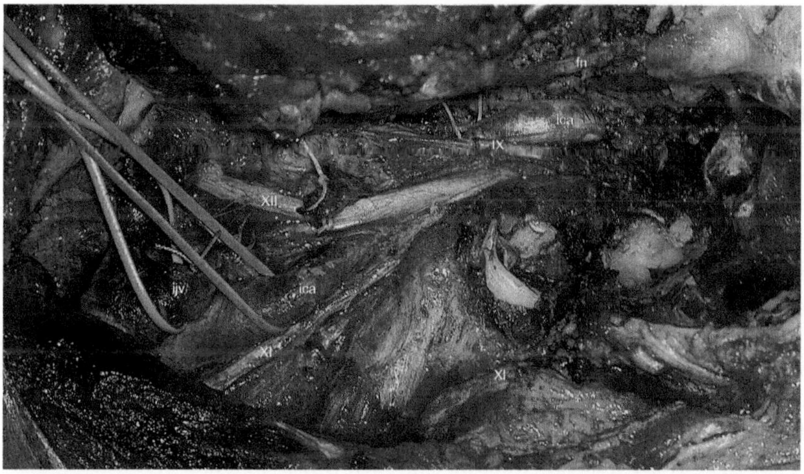

FIGURE 8.13

Type A Fisch infratemporal fossa approach, left side. Final view of the surgical field showing both the neck and the temporal sites. Due to the spread of the lesion to the internal carotid artery, the vessel was embolized before the surgical procedure, and it is shown as ligated and transected at the level of its horizontal tract. The internal jugular vein was also involved by the disease and it was resected in the neck. The facial nerve is shown transposed in the anterior portion of the field. *fa*, rerouted facial nerve; *ica*, internal carotid artery; *ijv*, internal jugular vein; *IX*, IX cranial nerve; *XI*, XI cranial nerve; *XII*, XII cranial nerve.

technique allows a good exposure of the IFT but the middle ear and Eustachian tube areas are not obliterated, the intratemporal facial nerve is not rerouted, and the petrous ICA is not fully exposed.

These approaches require an extensive bone and soft tissue demolition, and they are characterized by a large surgical field.

For the IFT approaches, exoscopic surgery is used both for the demolition of the temporal bone and the dissection of the neck at the level of the skull base, so for the isolation of vessels and nerves, for parotid gland dissection and for the isolation of the intraparotid facial nerve.

It can also replace the microscope in case of nerve anastomosis, for example, in the case of facial nerve dynamic reconstruction through end-to-end nerve anastomosis and cable graft interposition.

8.2.5.2 Retrolabyrinthine, translabyrinthine, transcochlear, transotic, transcanal transpromontorial approaches, subtotal petrosectomy

The transtemporal approaches are surgical procedures performed to reach the lateral skull base through the temporal bone.

In our experience, for the lateral approaches to the lateral skull base, the exoscope has proved to be an effective replacement of the operative microscope in the bone work, that is the demolition of the temporal bone to reach the most frequent pathological processes of the lateral skull base, such as petrous bone cholesteatomas and acoustic neuromas.

The choice of the approach depends on the histology, the preoperative hearing facial functions, and the localization and extension of the lesion to be tackled.

Among these approaches, the translabyrinthine approach is the most widely used by neurotologists (Figs. 8.14–8.17).

Here, the use of the exoscope during the labyrinthectomy has shown to be comparable to the microscope. However, through the translabyrinthine route, the intradural work in the CPA and the exposure of the anatomical structures in this area may not be the best ones, as the light of the exoscope cannot fully illuminate the field. Thus, it is worth using a translabyrinthine approach with an exoscopic view in case of a schwannoma involving the internal auditory canal with minimal extension to the CPA. Conversely, if a schwannoma has a substantial extension to the CPA, we recommend the use of an enlarged translabyrinthine approach with transapical extension that allows for a wider and better working area at the level of the CPA to obtain a good exposure of the structures in this area.

In the transcanal transpromontorial approach, the surgical corridor on the CPA is narrower than in the translabyrinthine approach (Figs. 8.18 and 8.19).

In this case, the exoscope can be used during the first steps of the dissection, except for the CPA because the corridor does not allow a good exposure, so a microscopic assistance is necessary for tumor dissection in the CPA.

In fact, a large surgical route is crucial for exoscope use. The best exoscopic use occurs during more extended and "enlarged" transtemporal approaches such as the transotic and transcochlear corridors, where the exposure of the intradural

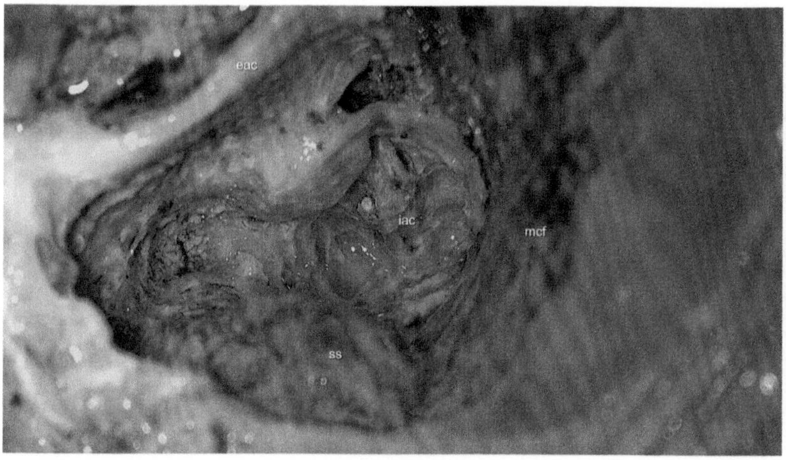

FIGURE 8.14

Translabyrinthine approach, left side. A mastoidectomy has been performed and the classic anatomical landmarks are in view (the sigmoid sinus, the middle cranial fossa dura ad the posterior wall of the external auditory canal). Moreover, a labyrinthectomy has been carried out and the internal auditory canal has been skeletonized. *eac*, posterior wall of external auditory canal; *iac*, internal auditory canal; *mcf*, middle cranial fossa; *ss*, sigmoid sinus.

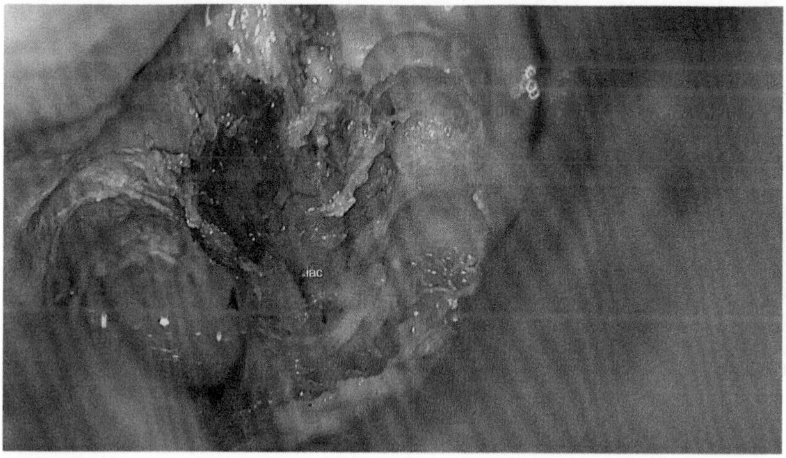

FIGURE 8.15

Translabyrinthine approach, left side. Zoomed view of the previous image, the internal auditory canal is center stage, the bone canal surrounding it has been furtherly drilled, and the dura of the canal is exposed. *iac*, internal auditory canal.

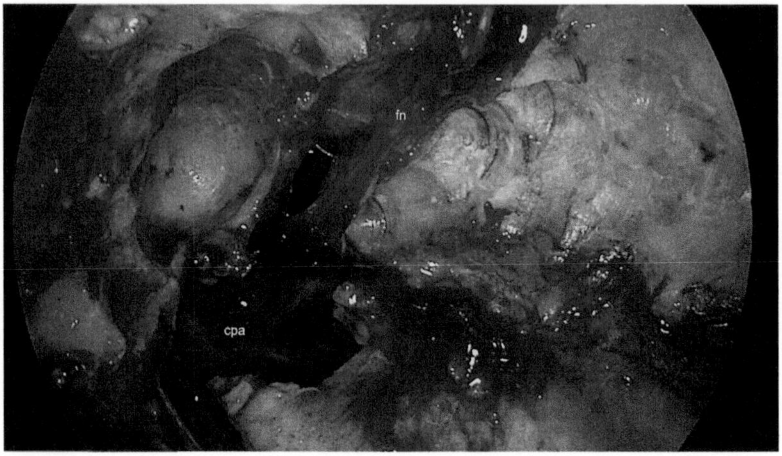

FIGURE 8.16

Translabyrinthine approach, left side. Endoscopic view, the dura of the internal auditory canal has been opened, the intrameatal facial nerve is exposed, and a portion of the cerebellar pontine angle is accessible. *cpa*, cerebellopontine angle; *fn*, intrameatal facial nerve.

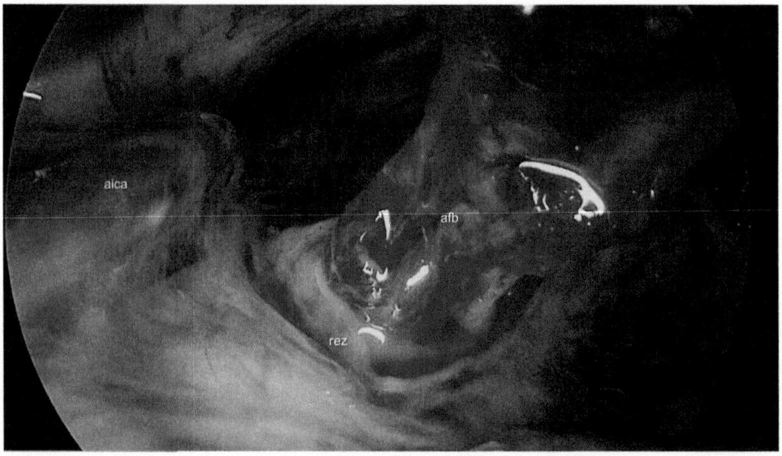

FIGURE 8.17

Translabyrinthine approach, left side. Endoscopic view, further magnification of the region of the cerebellar pontine angle, the acoustic facial bundle is in view, stemming from its entry zone in the pons. The anterior inferior cerebellar artery is shown too, soon after detaching from the basilar artery. *afb*, acoustic facial bundle; *aica*, anterior inferior cerebellar artery; *rez*, root entry/exit zone.

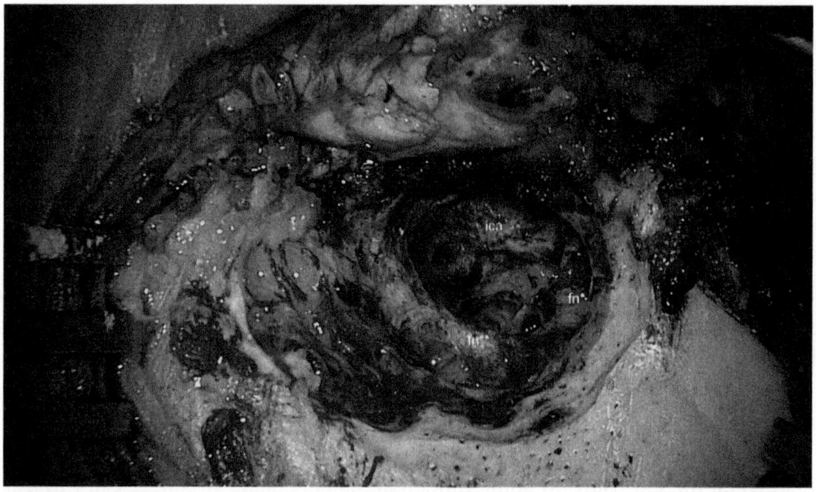

FIGURE 8.18

Enlarged transcanal transpromontorial approach, left side. View of the whole surgical corridor to access the internal auditory canal through this surgical procedure. The intrapetrous internal carotid artery and both the mastoid and the tympanic segment of the facial nerve can be seen. *fn**, tympanic segment of facial nerve; *fn***, mastoid segment of facial nerve; *ica*, internal carotid artery.

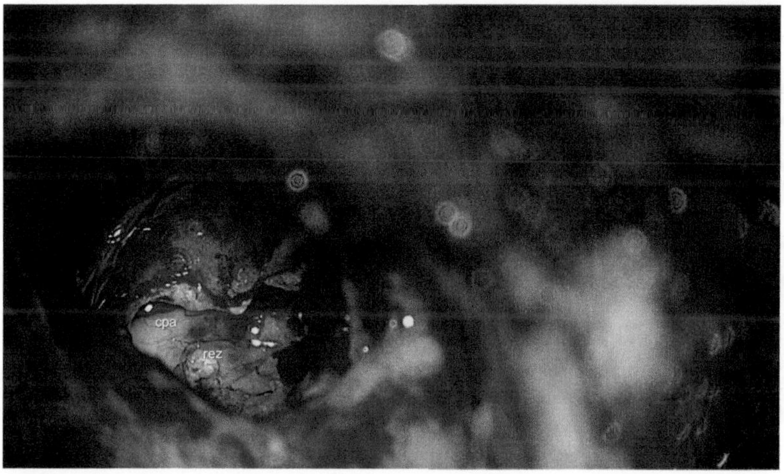

FIGURE 8.19

Enlarged transcanal transpromontorial approach, left side. In this approach, the narrow surgical corridor prevents the use of the exoscope for the access to the CPA, making the use of the microscope necessary. The promontory has been completely drilled away and the cerebellar pontine angle and the entry zone of the acoustic facial bundle are thus accessible. *cpa*, cerebellopontine angle; *rez*, root entry/exit zone.

anatomical structures becomes necessarily wider, allowing for a good illumination of the CPA also through exoscopy.

During the subtotal petrosectomy, all surgical steps can easily be replaced by the exoscope because all the anatomical structures are exposed without hidden areas.

8.2.5.3 Middle cranial fossa approach, anterior petrosectomy

The middle fossa approach is a useful option for small lesions of the internal auditory canal, when hearing might be preserved. The approach is versatile because it can be anteriorly extended by drilling the petrous apex (Kawase's triangle) and gaining access to the posterior fossa and petroclival area. For this kind of approach, the exoscope effectively replaces the microscope. However, a final endoscopic check to explore the blind areas like the fundus of the internal auditory canal, especially underneath the transverse crest, and the inferior portion of the horizontal tract of the internal carotid artery (Figs. 8.20–8.25).

The exoscope, like the operative microscope, has a direct view of the surgical field, so when the exposure of some hidden areas is needed, it is necessary to associate the use of an endoscope with angled optics, in particular, in the transotic approach, when surgical control medial to the tympanic and labyrinthine tracts of the facial nerve or medial to the vertical and horizontal tracts of the intrapetrous internal carotid artery is necessary.

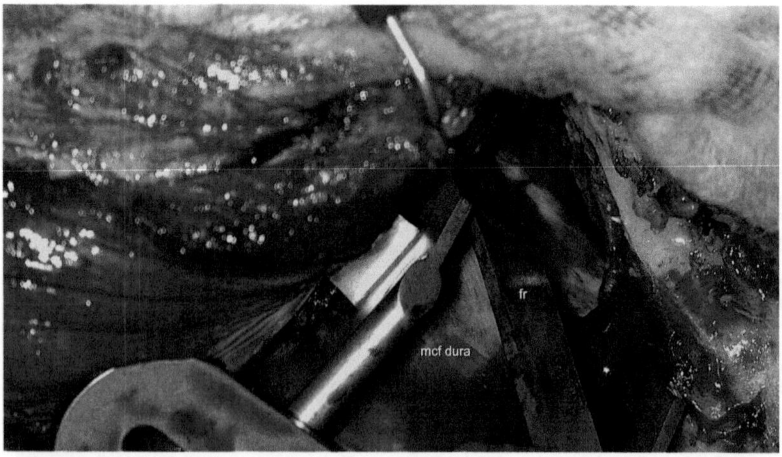

FIGURE 8.20

Middle cranial fossa approach, left side. Image showing the Fisch retractor that is used to expose the petrous bone by retracting the middle cranial fossa dura and the temporal lobe, thus creating an appropriate surgical field for this kind of approach. *fr*, Fisch retractor; *mcf dura*, dura mater of middle cranial fossa.

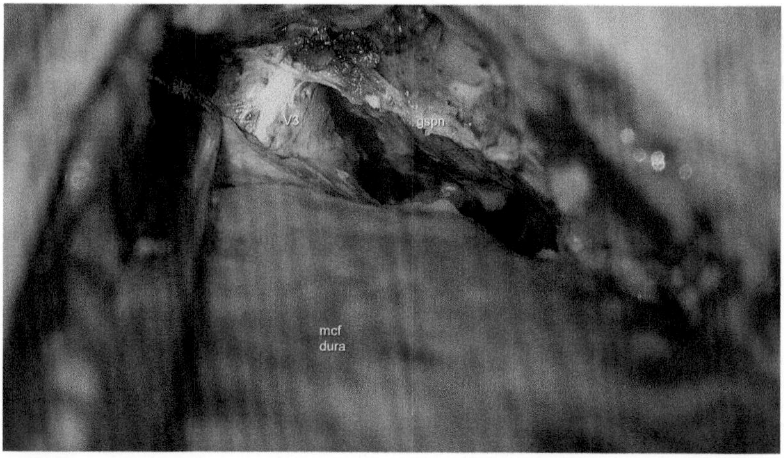

FIGURE 8.21

Middle cranial fossa approach, left side. This image shows the anterior portion of the surgical field, the mandibular division of the trigeminal nerve is shown as the anterior limit of the procedure while the middle meningeal artery has already been cauterized. The Greater petrosal nerve can also be spotted running just above the horizontal portion of the intrapetrous internal carotid artery. *gspn*, greater superficial petrosal nerve; *mcf dura*, dura mater of middle cranial fossa; *V3*, mandibular division of trigeminal nerve.

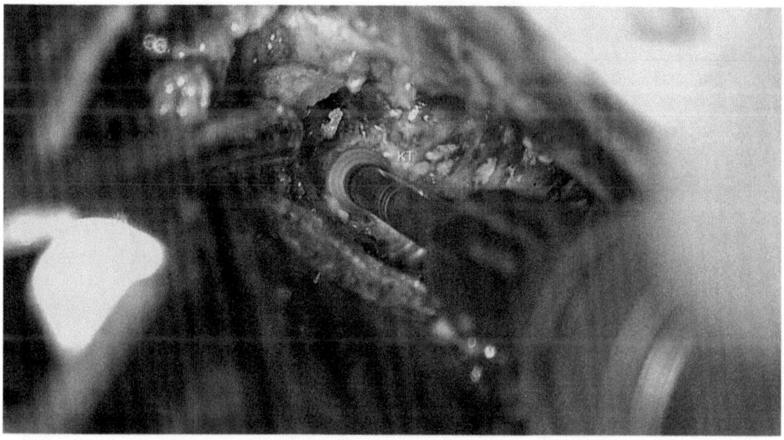

FIGURE 8.22

Middle cranial fossa approach, left side. The image allows to appreciate the surgical view during bone drilling. In this instance, the surgeon is working on the Kawase area whose boundaries are the junction of the greater superficial petrosal nerve with the lateral border of the mandibular division of the trigeminal nerve, the lateral margin of the porus trigeminus, and the anteromedial margin of the arcuate eminence. *KT*, kawase triangle (posteromedial triangle).

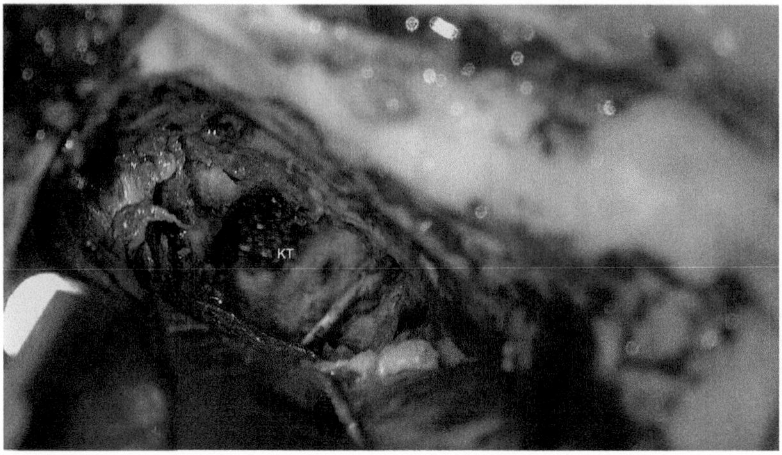

FIGURE 8.23

Middle cranial fossa approach, left side. The Kawase area has been completely drilled away. *KT, kawase triangle (posteromedial triangle).*

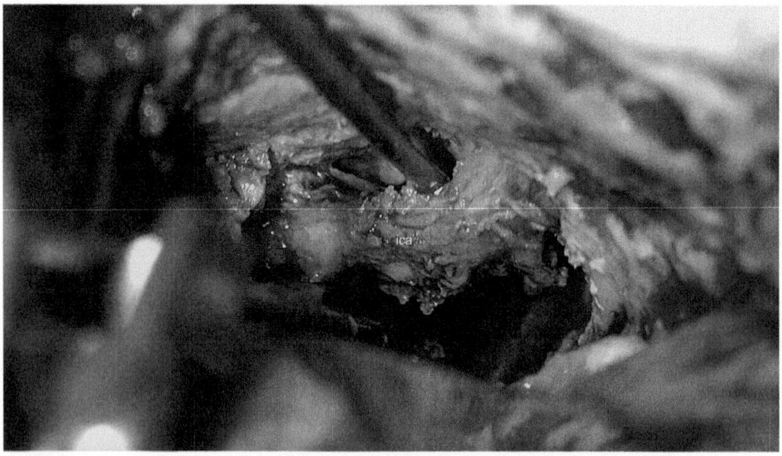

FIGURE 8.24

Middle cranial fossa approach, left side. The horizontal portion of the intrapetrous internal carotid artery has been totally skeletonized, allowing for a complete control of this delicate anatomical structure. *ica*, intarpetrous internal carotid artery (horizontal tract).

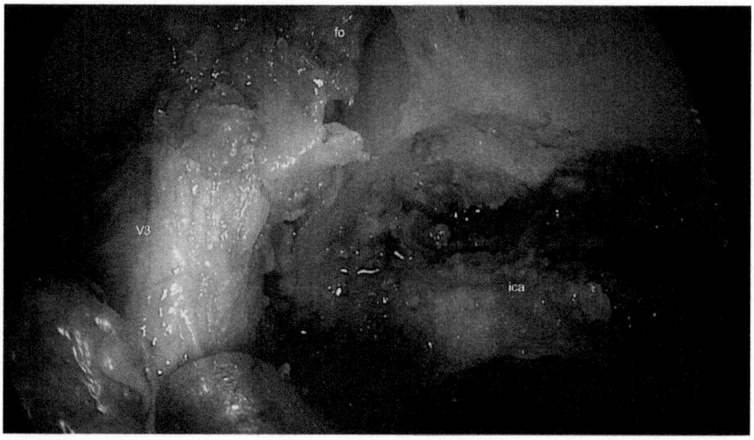

FIGURE 8.25

Middle cranial fossa approach, left side. Introducing the endoscope in the surgical field at this point grants a better visualization of the mandibular nerve, entering the foramen ovale, and the horizontal portion of the internal carotid artery, enabling additional surgical management of these landmarks. *fo*, foramen ovale; *ica*, intarpetrous internal carotid artery (horizontal tract); *V3*, mandibular division of trigeminal nerve.

8.3 Review of existing literature

3D exoscope has recently been introduced in daily clinical practice.

While for neurosurgery the effectiveness of this device is starting to be explored in literature, either as an exclusive instrument or in combination with a microscope, only very few studies have been carried out regarding otology and neurotology.

In the literature, image quality and definition have been considered similar between microscopic and exoscopic view.[3]

Furthermore, the minimal dizziness and discomfort, described using a 3D vision during surgery, are shown to be overcome as time goes by and through experience.[6]

Smith and colleagues showed that 3D exoscopes are potentially viable alternatives to the operating microscope for otologic and neurotologic procedures in particular for operations performed through relatively wide surgical apertures. They underlined some subjective advantages including superior ergonomics, compact size, and an equal visual experience for surgeons and observers. Their case series involved 11 patients where surgery was performed using a 3D exoscope to replace or in combination with the operating microscope. The exoscope was the sole visualization tool in seven cases, while four required the additional use of an endoscope or a microscope, no perioperative complications occurred and all cases were successfully completed.[5]

Garneau and colleagues described a cohort of six patients undergoing lateral skull-base surgery with the use of the exoscope for vestibular schwannoma resection (four cases) and for the repair of a temporal lobe encephalocele (two cases). They demonstrated the feasibility of the exoscope to perform all essential surgical maneuvers during both the transmastoid approach (mastoidectomy) and the transtemporal craniotomy along with the skull-base repair.

Never was it necessary to switch to microscopic view and all the operations were carried out without major complications.[7]

The current authors (D.M., A.R.) and colleagues carried out a retrospective study including 24 patients suffering from lateral skull-base pathologies who underwent surgery using either a 3D exoscope or an operative microscope. Both the exoscope and the microscope group included 12 cases. The two groups were compared considering surgical time, facial and hearing function outcomes, as well as intraoperative and postoperative complications.

No significant statistical differences were identified between them. Moreover, facial and hearing function outcomes were nearly equivalent. Also, the efficacy of a 3D exoscope in the different surgical steps on soft tissue, bone work, and tumor dissection was analyzed and demonstrated. In the literature, there are no studies in which a group of exoscopic procedures to the lateral skull base is compared to a control group of microscopic approaches both performed by the same surgeon (D.M.), and this is paramount to properly compare the two surgical visualization tools.[8]

References

1. Kwan K, Schneider JR, Du V, et al. Lessons learned using a high-definition 3-dimensional exoscope for spinal surgery. *Oper Neurosurg (Hagerstown)*. 2019;16(5):619–625. https://doi.org/10.1093/ons/opy196.
2. Sack J, Steinberg JA, Rennert RC, et al. Initial experience using a high-definition 3-dimensional exoscope system for microneurosurgery. *Oper Neurosurg (Hagerstown)*. 2018;14(4):395–401. https://doi.org/10.1093/ons/opx145.
3. Beez T, Munoz-Bendix C, Beseoglu K, Steiger HJ, Ahmadi SA. First clinical applications of a high-definition three-dimensional exoscope in pediatric neurosurgery. *Cureus*. 2018; 10(1):e2108. https://doi.org/10.7759/cureus.2108.
4. Rossini Z, Cardia A, Milani D, Lasio GB, Fornari M, D'Angelo V. VITOM 3D: preliminary experience in cranial surgery. *World Neurosurg*. 2017;107:663–668. https://doi.org/10.1016/j.wneu.2017.08.083.
5. Smith S, Kozin ED, Kanumuri VV, et al. Initial experience with 3-dimensional exoscope-assisted transmastoid and lateral skull base surgery. *Otolaryngol Head Neck Surg*. 2019; 160(2):364–367. https://doi.org/10.1177/0194599818816965.
6. Kong SH, Oh BM, Yoon H, et al. Comparison of two- and three-dimensional camera systems in laparoscopic performance: a novel 3D system with one camera. *Surg Endosc*. 2010;24(5):1132–1143. https://doi.org/10.1007/s00464-009-0740-8.
7. Garneau JC, Laitman BM, Cosetti MK, Hadjipanayis C, Wanna G. The use of the exoscope in lateral skull base surgery: advantages and limitations. *Otol Neurotol*. 2019; 40(2):236–240. https://doi.org/10.1097/MAO.0000000000002095.
8. Rubini A, Di Gioia S, Marchioni D. 3D exoscopic surgery of lateral skull base. *Eur Arch Otorhinolaryngol*. 2020;277(3):687–694. https://doi.org/10.1007/s00405-019-05736-7.

CHAPTER

The application of the exoscope in lacrimal surgery

9

Luca Malvezzi, MD [1,2], Francesca Pirola, MD [1,2]

[1]*Department of Biomedical Sciences, Humanitas University, Pieve Emanuele, Milan, Italy;* [2]*Otorhinolaryngology Unit, IRCCS Humanitas Clinical and Research Center, Rozzano, Milan, Italy*

9.1 Introduction

9.1.1 Anatomy and physiology of the lacrimal drainage apparatus

The lacrimal drainage apparatus is a system that carries tears, produced by the lacrimal gland, from the ocular surface to the nasal cavity.[1] It is defined by the following structures: the puncta, the canaliculi, the lacrimal sac, and the nasolacrimal duct. Moreover, two one-way valves are physiologically important to prevent tear reflux: the valve of Rosenmüller and the valve of Hasner (Fig. 9.1). Different mechanisms have been proposed to describe tear flow from the ocular surface to the nasal cavity, and the most relevant was theorized in 1960s and named "Jones' pump," from the name of the ophthalmologist who conceived it.[2]

As for the external oculo-lacrimal anatomy, full knowledge of the endonasal anatomy is fundamental. In particular, the lateral nasal wall in its most anterior part is the area of interest for lacrimal surgery. When introducing the endoscope into the nose beyond the nasal vestibule, the inferior and the middle turbinates are found laterally, inserting onto the lateral wall. In the inferior meatus localized below the inferior turbinate, we find the entrance to the nasolacrimal canal and the valve of Hasner. The middle meatus is below and lateral to the middle turbinate. The most important structures in this region are the uncinate process, the infundibulum with the hiatus semilunaris, and the ethmoidal bulla. In front of the superior insertion of the middle turbinate is the agger nasi, which represents the most anterior ethmoidal cell. Once these structures are recognized, the area that corresponds to the fossa where the lacrimal sac is located should be identified above the insertion of the anterior end of the middle turbinate. In particular, the major portion of the sac (approximately 10 mm) is found above the axilla of the middle turbinate.

9.1.2 Pathology

Disorders of the lacrimal drainage apparatus arise from abnormalities affecting any point along the tears passageway. Canalicular obstruction may be attributed to several etiologies, either congenital[3,4] (e.g., punctal atresia, canalicular obstruction,

Exoscope-Assisted Surgery in Otorhinolaryngology. https://doi.org/10.1016/B978-0-323-83168-0.00010-0

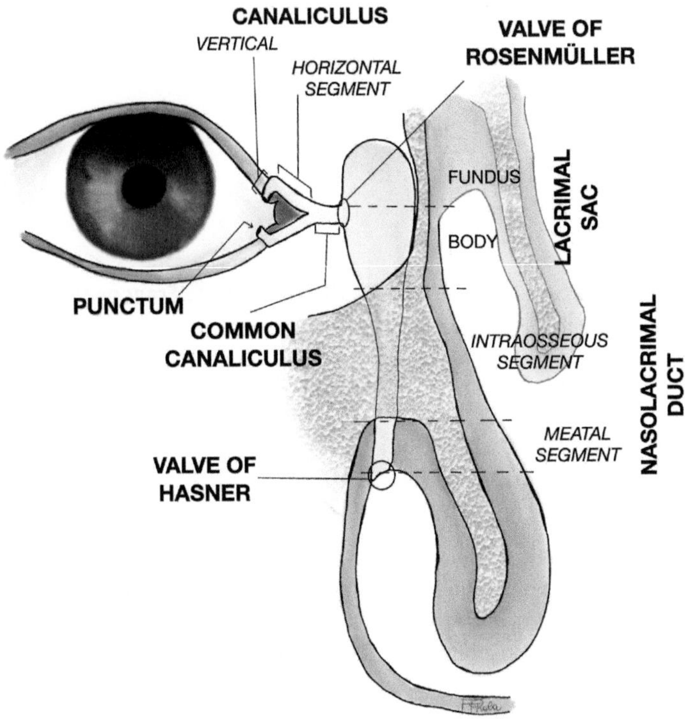

FIGURE 9.1

Anatomy of the lacrimal drainage apparatus.

common canalicular stenosis, in cases of anophthalmia or microphthalmia) or acquired. The latter ones may be inflammatory (e.g., blepharitis), traumatic (e.g., canalicular laceration or chemical burn), drug-induced (e.g., by taxanes or Mitomycin), iatrogenic (e.g., prior punctal plugs, punctal cauterization, postsurgical damage, longstanding lacrimal intubation, radiotherapy), or due to local malignancy.[5] However, most cases of lacrimal disorders are ascribable to abnormalities involving the nasolacrimal duct. Nasolacrimal duct obstructions (NLDO) may be classified as either congenital (CNLDO) or acquired. CNLDO is a common disorder in the pediatric population with a prevalence between 5% and 20% in early childhood,[6] causing impaired drainage of tears through the lacrimal system and clinically presenting with epiphora.[7] The acquired NLDO may be idiopathic (or primary), iatrogenic, or posttraumatic. The primary form is the most common, and its etiology is unknown. However, it is postulated that the primum movens for the occlusion of the lacrimal system is inflammation, even of unknown cause, that results in occlusive fibrosis and consequent epiphora.

Possible additional findings in adults are lacrimal sac mucocele or dacryocele/dacryocystocele (Fig. 9.2).[8] They refer to a dilated lacrimal sac that develops secondarily to the coexistence of a distal NLDO, and a proximal functional or

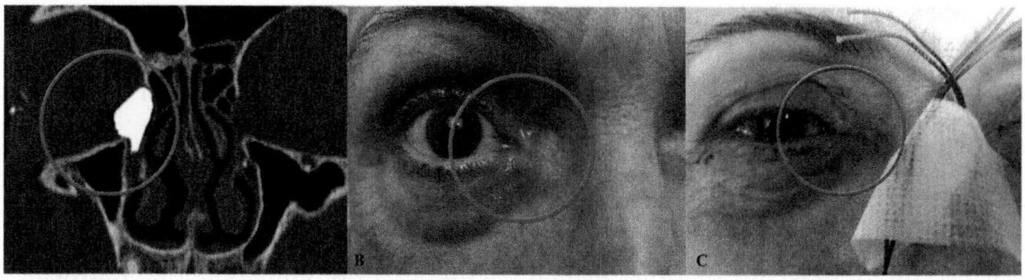

FIGURE 9.2

(A) Coronal dacryo-CT: in the red circle, contrast agent accumulation into the enlarged lacrimal sac (mucocele). (B) Preoperative external view of lacrimal sac mucocele. (C) Immediate postoperative external view of the same patient in B; reduction of the canthal region bulging is clearly visible.

structural obstruction (at the junction of the common canaliculus and lacrimal sac). It commonly presents as a mass in the medial canthal region accompanied by epiphora, and sometimes complicated by episodes of inflammation/infection (dacryocystitis/mucopyocele) (Fig. 9.3). Various hypotheses to describe its pathophysiology have been postulated, with two of them being the most accredited ones. A congenital or acquired (due to inflammation or trauma) obstruction of the distal NLD may cause secretions to accumulate within the sac. The increasing pressure on the sac walls may reach the area of junction between the sac and the two canaliculi, causing them to fold upon themselves and displace, resulting in proximal obstruction. The other postulated mechanism includes kinking of the common canaliculus due to malfunction of the Valve of Rosenmüller, that is the entrance of the common canaliculus into the lacrimal sac, secondary to edema and inflammation.

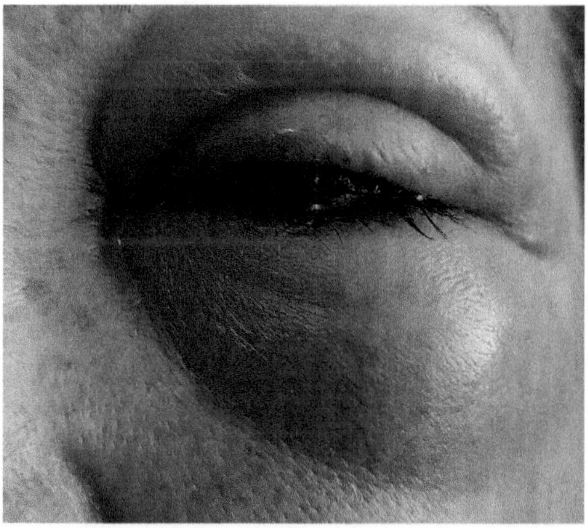

FIGURE 9.3

Mucopyocele of the left lacrimal sac with edema of the palpebral tissues.

Lacrimal sac mucoceles are known to cause bony erosion and remodeling, probably because of both inflammatory mediators and the pressure effect of the mass on the surrounding walls. Occasionally, this process extends to the overlying skin and spontaneous rupture or fistula formation may occur.

For what concerns treatments of pediatric CNLDO, conservative therapy (e.g., observation, lacrimal sac massage, and antibiotics) seem to be the best option in infants aged less than 1 year. On the other hand, in children older than 1 year, probing is successful for most obstructions, even if the timing for probing remains controversial and debated. In adult patients, surgery (e.g., dacryocystorhinostomy) is the gold standard treatment for acquired NLDO.

9.2 Operative techniques

9.2.1 Indications and contraindications

Indications to perform lacrimal surgery include cases of clinically significant epiphora or chronic conjunctivitis in the presence of nasolacrimal duct obstruction, recurrent dacryocystitis, or the presence of dacryoliths in the lacrimal sac that cause recurring episodes of nasolacrimal duct obstruction.

Malignancy of the lacrimal sac represents the only absolute contraindication to lacrimal surgery. Active dacryocystitis is a relative contraindication to the ab externo approach (see Section 9.2.2).

9.2.2 Different surgical approaches

Nowadays, different approaches are applied to manage conditions of the lacrimal drainage system. In particular, we find probing of the lacrimal way, balloon dacryoplasty, and ab externo dacryocystorhinostomy (DCR) as surgical alternatives to endoscopic DCR.

9.2.2.1 Probing and irrigation

Probing of the lacrimal way and irrigation is typically insufficient to resolve obstruction in adults, but it may be effective in pediatric cases of NLDO that do not resolve spontaneously or have an incomplete resolution after medical conservative therapy.[9] In cases of recurrent NLDO in which probing was not successful, balloon dacryoplasty or DCR may need to be performed.

9.2.2.2 Balloon dacryoplasty

Some authors consider performing balloon dacryoplasty for adult patients with incomplete obstruction ($\leq$50%), with a success rate varying from 20% to 90%. The procedure consists of dilating the puncta and inserting a Bowman probe. Then, a 3-mm balloon catheter is introduced into the nasolacrimal canal. Once a specific length mark is encountered, the balloon is inflated to a certain pressure and for a certain amount of time. The same inflation is made at precise points as the catheter is progressively retracted.

9.2.2.3 Ab externo DCR

Ab externo DCR is another approach to create a new passageway for tears into the nose. Surgery can be performed under general anesthesia or local-regional anesthesia with sedation (supratrochlear and infraorbital regional blocks may also be used). A vertical incision of approximately 10 mm is made anteriorly to the medial canthus. Then, dissection is carried out till the periosteum and the superficial head of the medial canthal tendon are reached and elevated. The lacrimal sac is encountered, and the fossa is exposed to find the line of the maxillolacrimal bone junction. This is the site of weakness where the bony ostium is created, either by expressing with the periosteal elevator to fracture the bone inward or by using chisel and mallet. The osteotomy is then enlarged up to approximately 10–15 mm in size. Afterward, the lacrimal sac posteromedial wall is tented with a Bowman probe, and it is incised and partially removed. y Nasal mucosa flaps are fashioned and sutured with the anterior sac wall to create the final rhinostomy. The skin is then closed with an interrupted suture, and silicon stents are positioned.

9.2.2.4 Endoscopic DCR

9.2.2.4.1 Evolution of the technique over the years

Endoscopic DCR operation has more than a century-long history. In 1893, Caldwell first described its endonasal approach, while a few years later Toti (1904) published the abovementioned external approach. The latter was initially adopted by the most, as the intranasal anatomy was dominated with difficulties and only poor instrumentation was available. Afterward, the technique varied a lot with the introduction of flaps during the 1920s and lacrimal stenting in the 1960s. During the last decades, the microscope that some authors used was progressively replaced by the endoscope, which was meanwhile grabbing the scene in nasal surgery. At that time, McDonogh and Meiring (1989) described the first modern endonasal DCR. Moreover, the application of argon laser for osteotomies increased over the 1990s. The external way had overall higher success rates (above 90%) and was indeed the preferred one. The application of the endonasal approach increased after endoscopes were introduced, and surgeons became more and more accustomed to them. Nowadays, endoscopic DCR is the standard approach recommended in the ENT field. It established its significance as a comparable technique to external DCR over the years, in terms of controlling lacrimal sac infections (dacryocystitis) and epiphora, with an average success rate of 87%.[10] Compared to the ab externo approach, endonasal DCR has multiple advantages: it avoids the risk of unacceptable cutaneous scarring; it has lower infection rates; it has the potential of prompt intervention in cases of mucopyocele. Some studies showed its additional and superior results to external DCR in the control of epiphora because of sparing Jones lacrimal pump, the periorbital muscular tissue, the skin, and surrounding structures. Moreover, a tailored access to the lateral nasal wall can be adopted in endoscopic DCR, allowing greater precision and bone preservation of the lateral wall anatomy, or concomitant correction of nasal bone variants if sinonasal pathology is present.

Over time, techniques in endonasal endoscopic DCR have changed. However, which one is the most effective is still debated. Novel approaches include the following: the use of nasal mucosal flaps after wide resection of bone; the direct milling of the lacrimal bone without the preparation of flaps; the use of lasers, drills, and/or scalpels. On the other hand, whether an anterior or a posterior approach to the lacrimal sac should be preferred is still a very active matter of debate.[11]

9.2.2.4.2 Description of the technique

In endoscopic DCR, lacrimal structures are approached from the inside of the nose, using endoscopes and sinonasal surgical instruments. The surgical technique that is mostly utilized worldwide is based on the one described by Wormald.[12] However, we have performed some modifications of the standard procedure in our experience. In fact, we do not perform the osteotomy of the frontal process of the maxilla or the preparation of nasal mucosal flaps. The purpose is always a wide marsupialization of the lacrimal sac onto the lateral nasal wall. The endoscope initially used is a camera with a 4-mm 0 degrees rigid optic. The surgical procedure starts with positioning nasal cottonoids with decongestant drugs in the middle meatus of the affected nostril. The first surgical step is retrograde uncinectomy with backbite forceps to show the natural ostium of the maxillary sinus. The vertical portion of the uncinate process is removed to give access to the lacrimal bone, and the cranial opening of a pneumatized agger nasi cell allows a clearer surgical field. The ophthalmologist introduces a light probe through the inferior lacrimal canaliculus, projecting onto the lateral nasal wall. The point of greatest luminescence corresponds to the least thick bone, that is the lacrimal bone. The area is drilled till the lacrimal sac is exposed with a high-speed diamond burr. According to this technique, the preparation of mucosal flaps is not necessary as the sac is exposed posteriorly to the frontal process of maxilla. The residual bone fragments are gently removed with pediatric Blakesley-Weil forceps. At this point, a rigid 4-mm 45 degrees endoscope is used. The lacrimal sac is tented and medialized by the ophthalmologist, producing a gentle pressure on the medial sac wall with the lacrimal probe. The sac is incised and its walls marsupialized with an angled scalpel and a circular cutting punch to expose the sac posterior aspect. The stoma must be as wide as possible to prevent its physiological partial retraction, and it is equally important to limit the exposure of bone surrounding the stoma to avoid excessive scarring. The lacrimal passageway is repeatedly washed with saline solution, then O'Donoghue lacrimal tubes are placed via the canaliculi and tied inside the nasal fossa. At the end of the procedure, one small cotton pattie is placed in the middle meatus for hemostatic purposes and removed at the patient's dismissal, which occurs 4 h after awakening from general anesthesia in a day-hospital setting. The entire surgery usually lasts about 20 min and has a comparable success rate to the ab externo technique (85%—90%), if performed on one side by an experienced surgeon and without the need of accessory sinonasal functional surgery).

Despite showing lower results in terms of outcomes (success rate of 77%), some surgeons have been recently employing a semiconductor diode laser in endoscopic

DCR to create the rhinostomy. This method is certainly faster, but it shows worse results than nonlaser endoscopic or external DCR at this time. Laser-assisted procedures very likely induce fibroblastic activity, thus excessive scarring and stenosis of the rhinostomy compared to the other techniques.

9.3 Exoscope-assisted lacrimal surgery

9.3.1 Introducing the exoscope into lacrimal surgery: considerations

Since January 2019, we have introduced the exoscope (VITOM 2D/3D by Karl Storz, Tuttlingen, Germany) in our operating room when performing lacrimal surgery.[13] It is a compact video microscope with 4K-resolution view and 3D technology, kept upon the surgical field by a specific holder (VERSACRANE), while displaying images on a screen. Provided with digital zooming, it can enlarge images up to 8–30 times, when held at a 20–50 cm distance over the surgical field. Moreover, thanks to exoscope's integrated control unit, recordings of procedures can be taken with very high quality (see also Chapter 1).

In our experience, proficient rhinologic surgeons performed more than 580 procedures (F = 78%, age range 17–84) over a period of 15 years, always in collaboration with ophthalmologists experienced in the field of lacrimal disorders. The exoscope has been introduced into lacrimal surgery with success during the last 18 months. More than 40 procedures were performed by the same experienced surgeons at this time, and an overall approval of this new instrument was obtained.[14] Despite much debate around the best technique to perform DCR, according to the authors, greater interest should be given in enhancing the collaboration between the ophthalmologist and the otolaryngologist, both in the operating room and during the entire diagnostic-therapeutic management of patients with lacrimal system pathology.

The exoscope was initially adapted in the field of lacrimal surgery thanks to its power of image magnification. In particular, a demanding step performed by the ophthalmologist is the correct intubation of the lacrimal way during the procedure: the surgeon—who is not wearing magnifying loops—may need to move close to the patient's eye for an easier viewing of the lacrimal punctae to perform intubation. This requires great visual efforts and sometimes longer time, if dealing with very small structures, especially in scarcely lit fields. Moreover, the operating room is usually dark during endoscopic procedures, and scialytic lights are used to a minimum. A possible remedy would use the endoscope as a source of light and magnification of the ocular area. However, this often does not prove to be satisfying, and it illogically binds the endoscope out of the nasal cavity. In this setting, the exoscope increases lightning (thanks to the camera light) only over the ocular area. Moreover, it magnifies field dimensions on the screen with excellent quality and without the unnatural rounded-shaping deformation usually caused by endoscopes (Fig. 9.4).

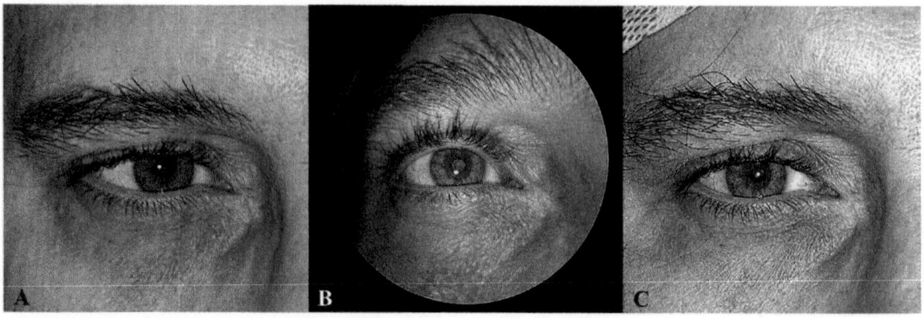

FIGURE 9.4

Outer ocular field. Comparison of pictures taken with a phone camera (A), with the endoscope (B), and with the exoscope (C).

Another noticeable and appreciated value of the exoscope is the simultaneous picture-in-picture (PiP) view: the screen is divided into two halves, one showing the intranasal structures (endoscopic view) and the other showing the outer ocular field (exoscopic view). This allows for better precision in lacrimal intubation and greater control of the probe direction, which can be extremely relevant in lowering the risk of undesirable false paths, especially if less experienced surgeons are performing their first DCR procedures. Additionally, it is worth mentioning that the PiP view is able to enhance intraoperative and postoperative teaching. In fact, operators and everyone else in the operating room are looking at the same screen, having the same visual inputs. In particular, in a study conducted upon attending trainees, it was reported that their visualization of the procedures was significantly upgraded, their understanding increased, and the teaching environment was boosted. Surgeons can explain phases of procedures just by referring to what anyone sees on the screen with the PiP view, even in the network connection. On the other hand, the ophthalmologist movements cannot be shown or recorded in DCR cases where the exoscope is not available. Finally, thanks to high-quality video documentation, footage can be used for later teaching or for reviewing critical steps of the operations to prepare for future cases. Although the educational advantage of exoscopic technology may be beneficial, further data are still needed to corroborate this aspect.

As previously mentioned, the collaboration between the ENT surgeon and the ophthalmologist is fundamental. The simultaneous view of the field on the split screen allows them to operate synchronously. The PiP view permits them not to move their head from their operating position (i.e., looking at the screen), as the other surgeon's movements are quickly visible at a glance (Fig. 9.5). Finally, another interesting value of the exoscope that might be considered is the fact that leaving the direct-vision traditional surgery toward an indirect-vision operating modality (through screens) might be a worthy training for surgeons, especially for ophthalmologists. Practicing with different sensory inputs increases functional plasticity, and it might eventually determine the surgeon's improvement in manual skills, as well as acquirement of new visual abilities and awareness.

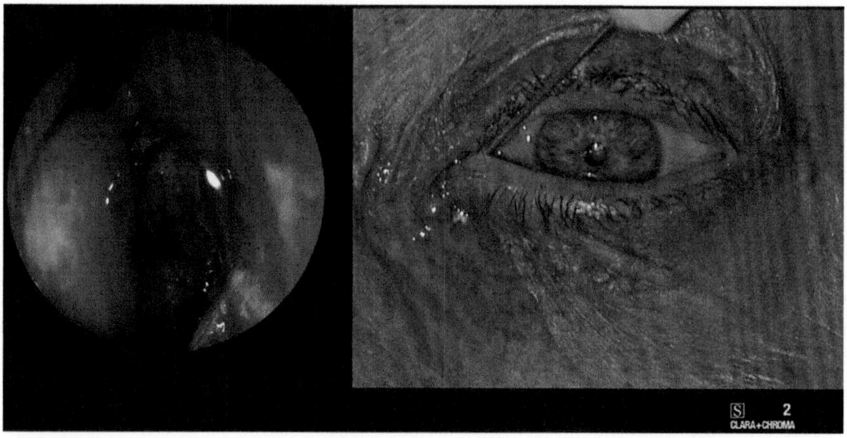

FIGURE 9.5

Split screen: simultaneous view of the endoscopic image (on the left) and the exoscopic one (on the right). Light probe inserted into the lacrimal way, showing the corresponding endoscopic position of the lacrimal sac.

9.3.2 Positioning the exoscope into the operating room

In lacrimal surgery procedures, the exoscope holder is placed behind one of the two surgeons (usually behind the ENT surgeon), with its arm holding the exoscopic camera that is leaning over the ocular field from below (Fig. 9.6).

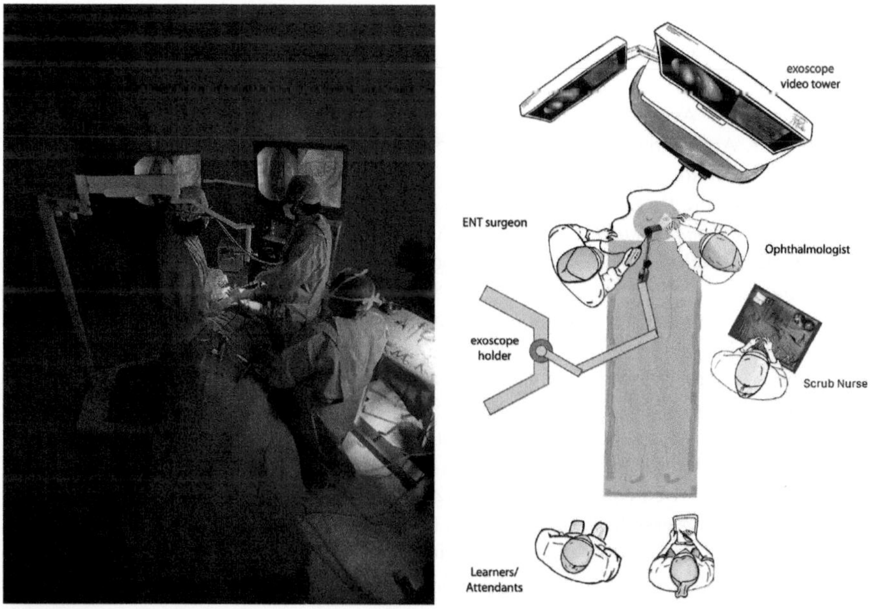

FIGURE 9.6

Setting of the operating room.

The video column is positioned at the head of the surgical bed with screens and recording unit. The two screens show the same images, and each one of them is set to face one surgeon so that they do not need to move from a natural and comfortable operating position. The scrub nurse is located behind the Ophthalmologist and is able to both see the screens and coordinate with the surgeons to hand them the surgical instruments.

9.3.3 Limitations about exoscope-assisted DCR

Despite approval and great utility of the exoscope in DCR, as previously depicted, some limitations may be found. First, a larger space is needed to comfortably place the equipment in the operating room, and to find the correct distance between the surgeons and the video column (for the best visual conditions and the least eye strain) is initially difficult. However, it must be considered that these drawbacks are often managed with time and experience, as proven in our practice. Another possible limitation is the cost of the machinery (VITOM exoscope, holder, video tower) if purchased only for nasal surgery. Nevertheless, it is a tool that is widely shared with other scenarios in the field of Otolaryngology and Head and Neck surgery (e.g., otosurgery, laryngeal microsurgery, and microvascular anastomosis in reconstructive surgery) and with other specialties inside hospitals and clinics (e.g., neurosurgery, vascular surgery). This is the case in which its costs become largely amortizable and its availability is able to bring interesting fallouts.

References

1. Cochran ML, Aslam S, Czyz CN. Anatomy, head and neck, eye nasolacrimal [Updated 2020 Jul 27]. In: *StatPearls [Internet]*. Treasure Island (FL): StatPearls Publishing; January 2020. Available from: https://www.ncbi.nlm.nih.gov/books/NBK482213/.
2. Jones LT. An anatomical approach to problems of the eyelids and lacrimal apparatus. *Arch Ophthalmol*. 1961;66:111–124.
3. Jones LT, Wobig JL. Congenital anomalies of the lacrimal system. In: *Surgery of the Eyelids and Lacrimal System*. Birmingham, AL: Aesculapius; 1976:157–173.
4. Sevel D. Development and congenital abnormalities of the nasolacrimal apparatus. *J Pediatr Ophthalmol Strabismus*. 1981;18:13–19.
5. Krishna Y, Coupland SE. Lacrimal sac tumors–a review. *Asia Pac J Ophthalmol (Phila)*. 2017;6(2):173–178.
6. Vagge A, Ferro Desideri L, Nucci P, et al. Congenital nasolacrimal duct obstruction (CNLDO): a review. *Diseases*. 2018;6(4):96.
7. MacEwen CJ, Young JD. Epiphora during the first year of life. *Eye*. 1991;5:596–600.
8. Yip C, McCulley TJ, Kersten RC, Bowen AT, Alam S, Kulwin DR. Adult nasolacrimal duct mucocele. *Arch Ophthalmol*. 2003;121(7):1065–1066.
9. Pediatric Eye Disease Investigator Group, Repka MX, Chandler DL, et al. Primary treatment of nasolacrimal duct obstruction with probing in children younger than 4 years. *Ophthalmology*. 2008;115(3):577–584.e3.

10. Huang J, Malek J, Chin D, et al. Systematic review and meta-analysis on outcomes for endoscopic versus external dacryocystorhinostomy. *Orbit*. 2014;33(2):81–90.
11. Wormald PJ, Kew J, Van Hasselt A. Intranasal anatomy of the nasolacrimal sac in endoscopic dacryocystorhinostomy. *Otolaryngol Head Neck Surg*. September 2000;123(3): 307–310.
12. Wormald PJ. Powered endoscopic dacryocystorhinostomy. *Laryngoscope*. 2002;112(1): 69–72.
13. Pirola F, Spriano G, Malvezzi L. Preliminary experience with exoscope in lacrimal surgery. *Eur Arch Otorhinolaryngol*. September 28, 2020. Epub ahead of print, PMID: 32989494.
14. Pirola F, De Virgilio A, Di Maria A, et al. Applying the exoscope to lacrimal surgery: preliminary experience. *ORL J Otorhinolaryngol Relat Spec*. 2021. *accepted, in print* 14539779074ne*n*..2.66.

CHAPTER

3D exoscopic parotidectomy

10

Roberto Puxeddu, MD, FRCS, Cinzia Mariani, MD, Valeria Marrosu, MD, Filippo Carta, MD

Unit of Otorhinolaryngology, Department of Surgery, Azienda Ospedaliero-Universitaria di Cagliari, University of Cagliari, Cagliari, Italy

10.1 Introduction

Benign parotid tumors have historically been treated by parotidectomy focused on the complete resection of the neoplasm with facial nerve preservation.[1]

Parotid masses were formerly managed via surgical enucleation, as first described by Beclard in 1824 with the aim of avoiding any facial nerve damage.[1,2] Nonetheless, tumor recurrence was pointed out in the mid-50s as the main risk of enucleation.[3] Since then, several modalities were used to treat patients with parotid tumors depending on the cytological nature and localization: extracapsular enucleation; removal of the tumor with a limited cuff of normal parotid tissue; superficial parotidectomy; subtotal resection of the parotid gland; and total parotidectomy.

Regardless of the indication for surgery and the nature of the lesions, parotidectomy is a challenging procedure requiring skilled surgeons due to the anatomical proximity of the facial nerve. The facial nerve identification itself is the key point in the outcome of this procedure, second only to the radicality of the resection.

Facial nerve identification can be achieved with two approaches: anterograde or retrograde dissection. It was advocated by Janes[4] and Bailey[5] to prior identify the main trunk of the facial nerve and subsequently to perform the parotidectomy. The anterograde approach allows the facial nerve identification at its emerge from the stylomastoid foramen. Using this technique, the reported recurrence rate and permanent facial nerve paralysis rate become very rare, decreasing to 0.2% and 2.2%, respectively.[6] In case of the lack of anatomical landmarks, revision surgery, or very bulging tumor, the detection of the main trunk of the facial nerve by an anterograde approach may be challenging. In such cases, the retrograde approach is crucial for nerve preservation avoiding spillage of the tumor. It consists of prior identification of a distal branch of the nerve and subsequently dissecting back to the main trunk.

Regardless of the nerve identification technique (whether anterograde or retrograde), its intraoperative preservation is supported by several tools such as loupes or the operative microscope. Although the loupes provide an excellent view,

Exoscope-Assisted Surgery in Otorhinolaryngology. https://doi.org/10.1016/B978-0-323-83168-0.00002-1

allowing for good dissection, the magnification is restricted to the surgeon unless coupled to a head microcamera. Microscope-assisted surgery offers high-intensity light and high magnification to the surgeon who works with a 3D view, but images are usually presented to the observers with 2D monitors with an unavoidable lack of depth-of-field information.[7]

The exoscope has been introduced as an alternative to a microscope in neurosurgery for 2D and, more recently, 3D viewing to overcome these limits.[8–12] It consists of a rigid rod lens video telescope that is suspended above the surgical field and displayed the image to a high-definition (HD) monitor in front of the surgeon (see Chapter 1). Recently, the use of 3D exoscopes has spread suitable for many surgical specialties such as gynecology, urology, and ENT. Thanks to the compact size and the high-quality images offered by the 3D-HD magnification, its use turned out to be ideal for parotid surgery, as reported in recently published preliminary experiences.[7,13]

10.2 Operating room setting

The operating room layout is configured to allow the surgeons to work closely to the surgical field and the scrub nurse to have an adequate range of movement to help the surgeons.

The 3D-HD exoscope (3D Vitom, Karl Storz, Tuttlingen, Germany) is positioned on the side of the first surgeon, approximately 30 cm from the surgical field. The main 55-in. 4K 3D monitor is positioned in front of the surgeon, at the eye level, while the second 3D monitor is oriented to allow the scrub nurse and assistants to have a good view (Figs. 10.1 and 10.2).

The surgeon is positioned on the left/right of the head of the patient (on the basis of the side of the lesion). The scrub nurse stands next to the first surgeon. The assistant stands at the patient's head, using the controller (IMAGE1 PILOT) covered with a sterile coating, to adjust the optical magnification and maintain the focus of the camera on the surgical field (Fig. 10.3). This position allows an easy view of the intraoperative nerve-monitoring device (Medtronic NIM Response 3.0), which is placed at the bottom of the surgical bed.

The use of polarized glasses is mandatory for all the theater attendants to perceive the 3D image.

10.3 Surgical technique

The surgical procedure is performed using the same surgical technique as in conventional parotid surgery, but the novelty is that the surgeon works with a direct vision to a 3D-HD 4K monitor, using polarizing eyeglasses, with a magnification of the anatomic structures from 8 to 30 times. The procedure is carried out under general

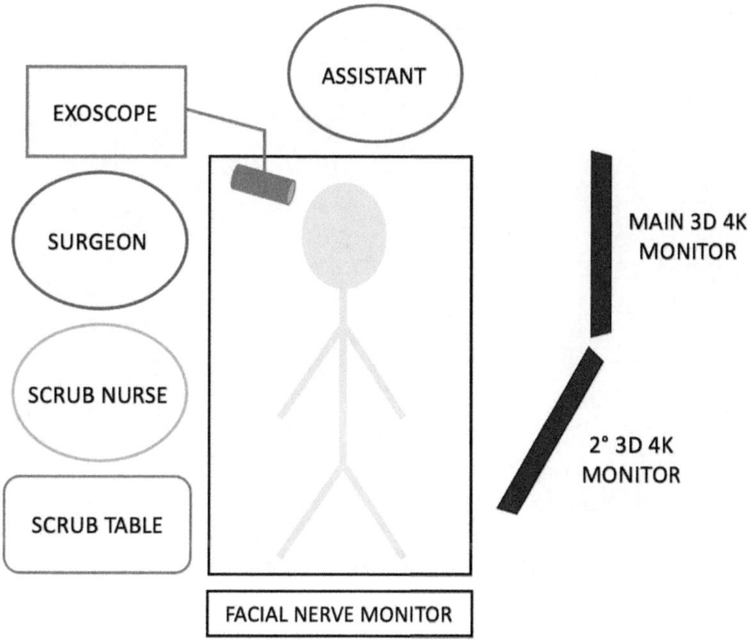

FIGURE 10.1

Theater setting scheme.

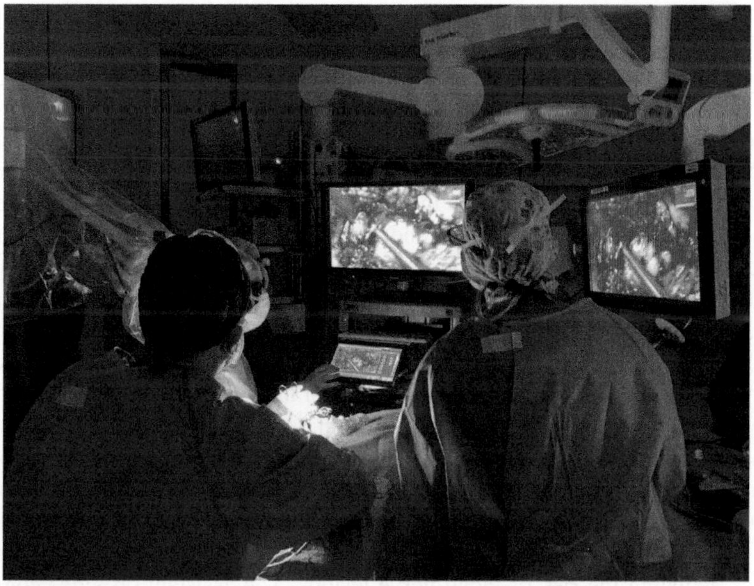

FIGURE 10.2

Monitor placement, allowing for a good view of all the surgical equipment.

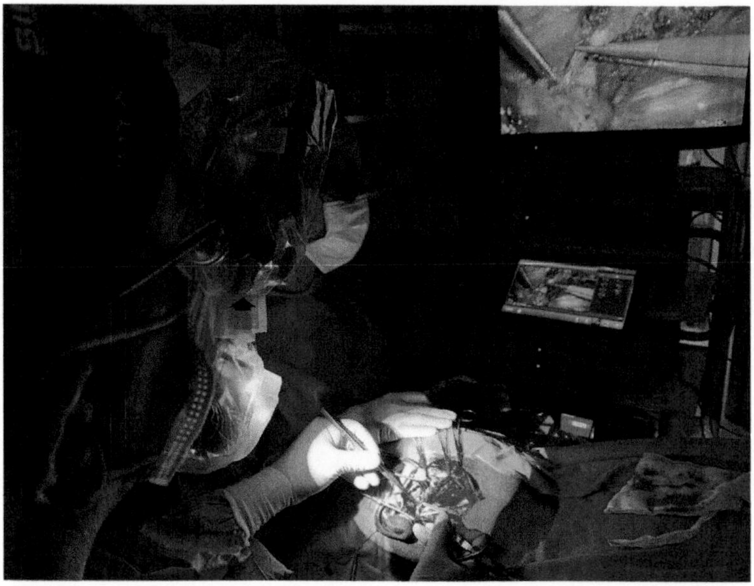

FIGURE 10.3

Assistant standing at the patient's head, using the controller (IMAGE1 PILOT) covered with a sterile coating, to adjust the optical magnification and maintain the focus of the camera on the surgical field.

anesthesia performed by nasotracheal intubation. The facial nerve function is monitored intraoperatively by a nerve integrity monitor (NIM) (Medtronic NIM Response 3.0 - 4 channels).

A modified Blair incision is usually performed, but a facelift incision can be preferred in selected cases. The anterior skin flap is elevated in the plane superficial to the parotid fascia. The great auricular nerve is preserved where possible to reduce the numbness of the auricular region in the postoperative period. The posterior belly of the digastric muscle is identified, and the parotid gland is mobilized from the tragal cartilage until the tragal pointer is reached. The main trunk of the facial nerve is identified where it emerges from the stylo-mastoid foramen, following the three classical landmarks: the tragal pointer, the tympano-mastoid suture, and the posterior belly of the digastric muscle. In selected cases in which the deepest aspect of the tumor is in wide contact with the main trunk of the nerve, a retrograde dissection of a peripheral facial nerve branch can be useful. Once the main trunk of the facial nerve is identified, it must be followed distally to the pes anserinus and the secondary branches, dividing the parenchyma that lies superficial to the nerve. Meticulous and blunt dissection of the peripheral branches is essential to avoid facial nerve injury. The use of the 3D exoscope allows for a great magnification of the finer branches, reducing the risk of facial nerve lesions. The assistant provides constant high-quality images, adjusting the magnification and maintaining the focus on the surgical field using the IMAGE1 PILOT.

The parotid tissue is progressively dissected free of the nerve until the superficial lobe is resected (type I–II parotidectomies according to the European Salivary Gland Society[14]). If the tumor is located in the deep lobe, after the resection of the superficial lobe, the procedure is extended by meticulous dissection of the main trunk and branches of the facial nerve from the underlying parotid tissue, until the deep parotid lobe is removed (type I–IV parotidectomies according to the European Salivary Gland Society[14]).

Thanks to the exoscope, the entire surgical team can benefit from the presence of 3D vision. In fact, it allows to directly experience all surgical steps, appreciating contextually all surgeon's fine gestures.

10.4 Outcomes

Eighteen cases of exoscopic parotidectomy have been reported in the literature so far[7,13] (Table 10.1).

Preoperative evaluations (both cytology and Magnetic Resonance Imaging) were indicative for benign lesions. In 17 patients (94.4%), the tumor was located in the superficial lobe, whereas in 1 case (5.6%) it arose in the deep lobe.

All the procedures were classified according to the European Salivary Gland Society[14]: one type I, eleven type I–II, five type II, and one type III.

The use of the 3D exoscope did not affect the operative time, allowing for a mean time of surgery of 147.2 min (range of 115–210 min).

There were no cases in which the operative staff needed to interrupt the 3D vision because of fatigue, headache, eye strain, dizziness, or other visually related problems. The postoperative period was free of complications for all the patients.

The 3D-HD magnification allowed for a minimally traumatic dissection of the facial nerve, because of the better understanding of the anatomic structures. The facial nerve was identified, carefully dissected, and preserved in all cases. No patient experienced definitive facial nerve palsy. One patient (5.6%) experienced postoperative transient grade II facial nerve deficit, as a consequence of adherence of the capsule of the tumor to the zygomatic branch of the nerve. In this case, the exoscopic view allowed for a precise dissection with no spillage of the neoplasm and a complete anatomic preservation of the nerve, with recovery within 3 months.[7]

Definitive histology confirmed the complete excision for all the specimens and the benign nature of the lesions: pleomorphic adenoma in 13 cases (72.2%) and Warthin's tumor in 5 cases (27.8%). These results show that 3D technology provides comparable radicality in the removal of benign parotid tumors, given that no cases of tumor spillage have been reported.

Table 10.1 Series of patients who underwent 3D exoscopic parotidectomy.

	Pt/sex/age	Localization	Surgical treatment	Operation time (min)	Postoperative facial nerve function	Other complications	Histology
Carta 2020[7]	1/F/47	Superficial lobe	Type I–II	145	Normal	No	Pleomorphic adenoma
	2/M/74	Superficial lobe	Type I–II	195	Normal	No	Pleomorphic adenoma
	3/M/60	Superficial lobe	Type I–II with retrograde facial nerve dissection	210	Normal	No	Pleomorphic adenoma
	4/M/65	Superficial lobe	Type I–II	170	Normal	No	Warthin's tumor
	5/F/33	Superficial lobe	Type I–II	120	Grade II	No	Pleomorphic adenoma
	6/M/48	Superficial lobe	Type I–II	115	Normal	No	Warthin's tumor
	7/M/42	Superficial lobe	Type I–II	135	Normal	No	Pleomorphic adenoma
	8/F/42	Superficial lobe	Type I–II	140	Normal	No	Pleomorphic adenoma
	9/M/19	Superficial lobe	Type I–II	115	Normal	No	Pleomorphic adenoma
Mincione 2020[13]	1/M/37	Superficial lobe	Type II	135	Normal	No	Pleomorphic adenoma
	2/M/59	Superficial lobe	Type I	138	Normal	No	Pleomorphic adenoma
	3/F/41	Superficial lobe	Type II	137	Normal	No	Pleomorphic adenoma
	4/M/68	Superficial lobe	Type I–II	142	Normal	No	Warthin's tumor
	5/F/28	Superficial lobe	Type II	148	Normal	No	Pleomorphic adenoma
	6/M/72	Deep lobe	Type III	165	Normal	No	Pleomorphic adenoma
	7/F/75	Superficial lobe	Type II	138	Normal	No	Warthin's tumor
	8/M/47	Superficial lobe	Type I–II	157	Normal	No	Pleomorphic adenoma
	9/F/61	Superficial lobe	Type II	145	Normal	No	Warthin's tumor

10.5 Advantages

The advent of 3D-HD exoscopes after the introduction of operative microscopes and endoscopes has enlarged surgical perspectives: these new optical devices present many features that can be considered as an evolution of magnified-assisted surgery.[7] The 3D technology provides enhanced depth perception, spatial orientation, image contrast, and color, with the possibility to apply light filters that can help to precisely identify the boundaries among lesion, vessels, nerves, and parenchyma.[13,15] The 3D magnification, stereoscopic vision, and 4K quality of the images allow for a blunt dissection of the finer branches of the facial nerve, reducing the risks of iatrogenic lesions. Furthermore, a radical excision appeared to be provided with magnification-assisted parotidectomy, granting optimal oncologic outcomes.[16–18]

The 3D-HD exoscope represents a valid alternative tool for magnification and lighting of the surgical field in parotid surgery that overcomes the limits of loupes and operative microscope. Binocular loupes have a fixed magnification from 2.5× to 5× and a fixed working distance that cannot be tailored according to the surgeon's preferences. In fact, it is not possible to increase the magnification, nor changing the work distance if needed intraoperatively. Moreover, excessive weight of the device or an incorrect working distance can predispose the surgeon to postures that may result in neck strain.[13] These issues altogether can burden the surgical outcomes, especially in challenging cases.

Despite the optimal view of the surgical field, the operative microscope constrains the location of the surgeon's eye and may force awkward postures, leading to neck and back pain, fatigue, and eye strain. In addition, preoperative settings and microscope positioning may be time consuming for less-skilled surgeons such as residents. Finally, the bulky dimension of the operative microscope limits the movement of both scrub nurse and assisting the surgeon during parotid surgery.

In a recent study by Yu et al.[19] examining the postural changes in microsurgical trainees on traditional stereoscopic microscopes versus a 3D video display, the authors observed that neck angles were more neutral on the video display compared to the microscope.[13,19] The exoscope allows for ergonomic work as the user is not confined to the eyepiece, and it enables improved workflow as all people in the surgical theater can view the procedure in the same image quality as the surgeon.[7] The possibility to enjoy a 3D perception of the surgical field, the anatomic details and the surgeon's fine gestures improves the learning process of residents and fellows. The educational potential of video displays is confirmed by the interactive feature provided by the IMAGE1 PILOT system. In fact, the assistant surgeon has to anticipate the moves of the first surgeon, changing the position on the operating field. For such reasons, the first operator needs to share all surgical gestures, precisely communicating with the assistant.

Furthermore, the possibility to record images in HD enables the surgeons to share videos for didactic sessions, webinars, and surgical courses,[20] even if image editing requires dedicated software.

Box 10.1 Take home messages

Key-Points:

- The 3D-HD exoscope technology enables surgeons to a precise surgical dissection of the parotid region with a real 3D magnification of the anatomical structures, with low risk for iatrogenic lesions of the facial nerve.
- The exoscope provides a more ergonomic work as the user is not confined to the eyepiece and enables improved workflow as all people in the surgical theater can view the procedure in the same image quality as the surgeon.
- The possibility to enjoy a 3D perception of the surgical field, anatomic details, and surgeon's fine gestures improves the learning process of residents and fellows.
- The educational potential of video displays is confirmed by the interactive feature provided by the pilot system: in fact, the surgical assistant has to anticipate first surgeon's moves, changing the focus and the framing of the operating field.

The main drawbacks of the 3D exoscopic surgery reported in the literature are asthenopia and the learning curve.[13] The eyestrain and associated symptoms such as nausea, vertigo, or headache have been related to an exaggerated mismatch of the binocular vision compared to the image fusional capacity of each individual.[21,22] However, the latest 3D monitors, including autostereoscopic displays and HD resolution, are designed to overcome the existing limitations.[22] Some authors reported that initial compliance to the new setting in terms of hand-eye coordination could be challenging, but ENT surgeons usually have a solid background in display-assisted procedures, both office-based and surgical.

Even though the surgeon's experience is the main factor for the surgical outcome in parotid surgery,[16] the preliminary applications of 3D-HD exoscopes in this specific surgical procedure showed promising results. The 3D-HD vision and the wide spectrum of magnification allowed a precise surgical dissection with low risk of iatrogenic lesion of the facial nerve, reducing the physical demands of microsurgery, allowing surgeons to select comfortable postures, and improving both team communication and teaching (Box 10.1).

References

1. Béclard PA. Extirpation de la parotide. *Arch Gén Méd.* 1824;4:60–66.
2. Coniglio AJ, Deal AM, Trevor MS. Outcomes of drainless outpatient parotidectomy. *Head Neck.* 2019;41(7):2154–2158. https://doi.org/10.1002/hed.25671.
3. Perzik SL. Parotid tumor operations; the case against enucleation. *Calif Med.* 1956;85(1): 26–29.
4. Janes RM. The treatment of tumours of the salivary glands by radical excision. *Can Med Assoc J.* 1940;43:554.

5. Bailey H. The treatment of tumours of the parotid gland with special reference to total parotidectomy. *Br J Surg*. 1941;28:337–346.
6. Foresta E, Torroni A, Di Nardo F, et al. Pleomorphic adenoma and benign parotid tumors: extracapsular dissection vs superficial parotidectomy - review of literature and meta-analysis. *Oral Surg Oral Med Oral Pathol Oral Radiol*. 2014;117(6):663–676. https://doi.org/10.1016/j.oooo.2014.02.026.
7. Carta F, Mariani C, Marrosu V, Gerosa C, Puxeddu R. Three-dimensional , high-definition exoscopic parotidectomy: a valid alternative to magnified-assisted surgery. *Br J Oral Maxillofac Surg*. 2020;58(9):1128–1132. https://doi.org/10.1016/j.bjoms.2020.06.015.
8. Birch K, Drazin D, Black KL, Williams J, Berci G, Mamelak AN. Clinical experience with a high definition exoscope system for surgery of pineal region lesions. *J Clin Neurosci*. 2014;21(7):1245–1249. https://doi.org/10.1016/j.jocn.2013.10.026.
9. Beez T, Munoz-Bendix C, Beseoglu K, Steiger H-J, Ahmadi SA. First clinical applications of a high-definition three-dimensional exoscope in pediatric neurosurgery. *Cureus*. 2018;10(1):1–8. https://doi.org/10.7759/cureus.2108.
10. Barbagallo GMV, Certo F. Three-dimensional, high-definition exoscopic anterior cervical discectomy and fusion: a valid alternative to microscope-assisted surgery. *World Neurosurg*. 2019;130:e244–e250. https://doi.org/10.1016/j.wneu.2019.06.049.
11. Garneau JC, Laitman BM, Cosetti MK, Hadjipanayis C, Wanna G. The use of the exoscope in lateral skull base surgery: advantages and limitations. *Otol Neurotol*. 2019; 40(2):236–240. https://doi.org/10.1097/MAO.0000000000002095.
12. Smith S, Kozin ED, Kanumuri VV, et al. Initial experience with 3-dimensional exoscope-assisted transmastoid and lateral skull base surgery. *Otolaryngol Head Neck Surg*. 2019; 160(2):364–367. https://doi.org/10.1177/0194599818816965.
13. Mincione A, Lepera D, Rizzi L. VITOM 3D system in parotid gland surgery. *J Craniofac Surg*. 2020;32(2):e138–e141. https://doi.org/10.1097/scs.0000000000006875.
14. Quer M, Guntinas-Lichius O, Marchal F, et al. Classification of parotidectomies: a proposal of the European Salivary Gland Society. *Eur Arch Otorhinolaryngol*. 2016; 273(10):3307–3312. https://doi.org/10.1007/s00405-016-3916-6.
15. Rossini Z, Cardia A, Milani D, Lasio GB, Fornari M, D'Angelo V. VITOM 3D: preliminary experience in cranial surgery. *World Neurosurg*. 2017;107:663–668. https://doi.org/10.1016/j.wneu.2017.08.083.
16. Carta F, Chuchueva N, Gerosa C, Sionis S, Caria RA, Puxeddu R. Parotid tumours: clinical and oncologic outcomes after microscope-assisted parotidectomy with intraoperative nerve monitoring. *Acta Otorhinolaryngol Ital*. 2017;37(5):375–386. https://doi.org/10.14639/0392-100X-1089.
17. Pia F, Policarpo M, Dosdegani R, Olina M, Brovelli F, Aluffi P. Centripetal approach to the facial nerve in parotid surgery: personal experience. *Acta Otorhinolaryngol Ital*. 2003;23(2):111–115.
18. Grosheva M, Klussmann JP, Grimminger C, et al. Electromyographic facial nerve monitoring during parotidectomy for benign lesions does not improve the outcome of postoperative facial nerve function: a prospective two-center trial. *Laryngoscope*. 2009; 119(12):2299–2305. https://doi.org/10.1002/lary.20637.
19. Yu D, Green C, Kasten SJ, Sackllah ME, Armstrong TJ. Effect of alternative video displays on postures, perceived effort, and performance during microsurgery skill tasks. *Appl Ergon*. 2016;53:281–289. https://doi.org/10.1016/j.apergo.2015.10.016.

20. Crosetti E, Arrigoni G, Manca A, Caracciolo A, Bertotto I, Succo G. 3D exoscopic surgery (3Des) for transoral oropharyngectomy. 2020;10(January):1–8. https://doi.org/10.3389/fonc.2020.00016.
21. Bang JW, Heo H, Choi JS, Park KR. Assessment of eye fatigue caused by 3D displays based on multimodal measurements. *Sensors (Switzerland)*. 2014;14(9):16467–16485. https://doi.org/10.3390/s140916467.
22. Molteni G, Nocini R, Ghirelli M, et al. Free flap head and neck microsurgery with VITOM R 3D: surgical outcomes and surgeon's perspective. *Auris Nasus Larynx*. 2020;48(3):464–470. https://doi.org/10.1016/j.anl.2020.09.010.

CHAPTER

11 Exoscope-assisted thyroid surgery

Giuseppe Mercante, MD [1,2], Andrea Costantino, MD [1,2], Francesca Gaino, MD [2]

[1]*Department of Biomedical Sciences, Humanitas University, Pieve Emanuele, Milan, Italy;*
[2]*Department of Otorhinolaryngology - Head and Neck Surgery, IRCCS Humanitas Research Hospital, Rozzano, Milan, Italy*

11.1 Technological advancements in thyroid and parathyroid surgery

At the beginning of the 21st century, technological advancements in thyroid and parathyroid surgery served to obtain better cosmetics results and lower postoperative pain. Minimally invasive video-assisted parathyroidectomy and thyroidectomy relied on the use of an endoscope.[1,2] A further upgrade was obtained by adding a three-dimensional (3D) view of the surgical field.[3] More recent techniques, including thyroidectomy via transaxillary approach,[4] transoral robotic-assisted thyroidectomy,[5] and transoral endoscopic thyroidectomy via vestibular approach,[6] rely on the use of endoscopes combined with 3D view. In fact, 3D vision allows for better identification and visualization of anatomical structures. Similar to previous endoscopic approaches, the exoscope combines 3D technology with 4K view and permits to perform thyroid surgery with an open approach, without changing surgical steps and using the same instrumentation, but resulting in enhanced vision.

The primary aim in thyroid surgery is to remove the gland tissue completely, while preserving the recurrent laryngeal nerve (RLN) and parathyroid glands (PGs). After a preliminary dissection, the RLN and PGs should be adequately identified and visualized to reduce the risk of iatrogenic damage. Although various medical devices have been developed for intraoperative use to simplify RLN and PGs identification, visual identification still represents the gold standard. Surgical loupes are widely used to enhance the surgical field magnification, reducing the risk of RLN tearing and PGs devascularization. However, the magnification is restricted to the surgeon unless the loupes are coupled to a microcamera. In this context, the introduction of the exoscope as a new visualization and magnification tool represents an innovative way to improve the identification and preservation of RLN and PGs during conventional open thyroidectomy. The exoscopic system projects the surgical image onto a 4K 3D 32-in. monitor that can be seen by all the operators and other surgical staff, allowing for an outstanding view of the surgical field, coupled with depth perception. Moreover, image magnification can be adjusted and modulated during the procedure to focus on anatomical structures of interest, aiding in surgical dissection.

Exoscope-Assisted Surgery in Otorhinolaryngology. https://doi.org/10.1016/B978-0-323-83168-0.00003-3

11.2 Exoscope configuration and setting for thyroid surgery

The Vitom exoscope, consisting of a telescopic 3D camera, with a magnification power of 8–30× and a depth of field of 7–44 mm, is connected to a 3D 4K resolution screen through the Image1 S platform. The operating camera is controlled by the Image1 Pilot, an intuitive joystick through which the surgeon can adjust zoom, focus, and other video settings during the procedure. The exoscope can be mounted on the Versacrane holding system, which can be manually adjusted by the operator to place the camera in the preferred position, allowing for a focal distance of 20–50 cm.

During thyroid surgery, the holding system is placed between the surgeon and assistant surgeon standing at the head of the patient, when three surgeons are performing the procedure. The exoscope is placed above the surgical field at a distance of approximately 40 cm. The Image1 Pilot is fixed to the surgical table and positioned toward the feet of the patient, between the surgeon and scrub nurse. Both the exoscope and the Image1 Pilot are covered in sterile drapes, allowing surgeons to move and adjust them during the procedure. The main screen is positioned in front of the first surgeon. Additional screens can be placed in the operating room, allowing assistant surgeons, scrub nurse, operating room staff, and observers to follow surgical steps. Those screens must be placed precisely in front of the intended user(s), to allow for a precise 3D visualization of the field. An example of the operating room setting is shown in Fig. 11.1.

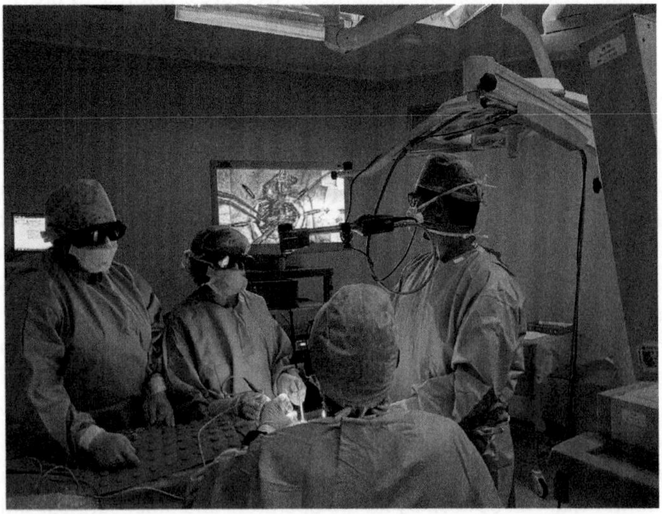

FIGURE 11.1

Operating room setting for exoscope-assisted thyroid surgery. Surgeons and scrub nurse wear 3D glasses and perform surgery looking at images projected on 3D screens.

11.3 Exoscope-assisted thyroid surgery

A midline neck incision is performed as in open conventional thyroidectomy. During the first part of the surgical operation, including skin incision, flap elevation, strap muscle dissection and superior vascular pedicle ligation, the exoscope is used only for didactic purposes, while it does not add a clear advantage to the surgical dissection. In particular, the first steps of the surgery involve the dissection of planes located at different depths and a wide surgical field, requiring continuous manual regulations of the exoscope, as adjustments with the Image1 Pilot are insufficient for clear focusing and zooming.

Once surgical landmarks (e.g., trachea, cricothyroid muscle) are adequately exposed, surgeons and scrubbed nurse wear 3D glasses and start using the exoscope, performing the following steps by screen visualization. At this stage, small vessels can be easily recognized and ligated to preserve the PGs. Once identified, the RLN is traced cephalad until it enters the cricothyroid membrane (Fig. 11.2). Then, the use of the exoscope is no longer mandatory, and the lobectomy could be then completed either with or without it. When central compartment neck dissection is performed, it can be conducted using the exoscope, in particular when the RLN is identified and separated from the lymph nodes along its course. Then, the exoscope is not strictly necessary, and the dissection could be completed on a direct vision. After lobectomy and ipsilateral central compartment dissection, the orientation of the image can be changed without moving the camera, and the same procedure is performed on the contralateral side. At the end of the procedure, hemostasis is performed with bipolar cautery under exoscopic vision to avoid nerve injury. The anatomic integrity of the RLN can be verified under exoscopic view before wound closure.

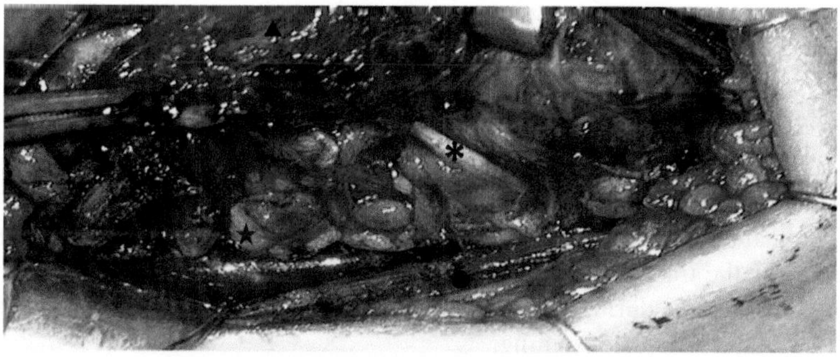

▲ thyroid gland, right lobe

✱ recurrent laryngeal nerve

● strap muscles

★ superior parathyroid gland

FIGURE 11.2

Anatomical landmarks identification during exoscope-assisted thyroid surgery.

11.4 Advantages of exoscope-assisted surgery in thyroid and parathyroid glands procedures

Exoscope-assisted surgery can be useful during open lobo-isthmusectomy, total thyroidectomy, and central compartment neck dissection, as well as in parathyroidectomy. The implementation of surgical field magnification by the exoscopic system improves the ability to perform precise dissection of fine structures. In particular, this technology could simplify the identification of RLN and PGs preservation. Although the exoscope was developed to substitute the operating microscope in microsurgical procedures, several papers have been recently published demonstrating the usefulness of exoscope-assisted open surgery. In particular, the exoscope was used for parotid surgery[7] and upper airway stimulation[8] during the identification and dissection of the facial and hypoglossal nerves, respectively.

Interestingly, this system provides the possibility to share the same vision of the main surgeon with operating room staff and observers during the procedure. In particular, the scrub nurse can benefit from the 3D vision on the 4K screen to better understand surgical steps and to anticipate the surgeon's next choice of instrument. The optimal ergonomics of the small 3D camera, associated with the slim holding system, allow for exoscope placement above the surgical field without interfering with surgical maneuvers. In addition, both the 3D camera and Image1 Pilot can be equipped with sterile covers, allowing autonomous adjustments during the operation without the need for dedicated staff. Additionally, the exoscope system offers the possibility to modulate the image magnification dynamically during the procedure. The ease of use of the joystick allows to move the camera and magnify the area of interest during the procedure assisting the surgeon during fine dissection. This represents an advantage compared to surgical loupes given their defined magnification that could not be easily changed during the procedure.

11.5 Pearls and pitfalls

- It is advisable that the first surgeon is seated during the surgical steps performed with the exoscope.
- The surgical table should be rotated 15–20 degrees away from the first surgeon to better focus the tracheoesophageal groove during RLN identification.
- Using the exoscope during steps not involving the identification/isolation of RLN and PGs may be time consuming.

References

1. Miccoli P, Berti P, Conte M, Raffaelli M, Materazzi G. Minimally invasive video-assisted parathyroidectomy: lesson learned from 137 cases. *J Am Coll Surg*. 2000;191(6): 613–618.
2. Miccoli P, Berti P, Raffaelli M, Conte M, Materazzi G, Galleri D. Minimally invasive video-assisted thyroidectomy. *Am J Surg*. 2001;181(6):567–570.
3. Mercante G, Battaglia P, Manciocco V, Cristalli G, Pellini R, Spriano G. Three-dimensional minimally invasive video-assisted thyroidectomy: preliminary report. *J Exp Clin Cancer Res*. 2013;32(1):78.
4. Kang SW, Jeong JJ, Yun JS, et al. Gasless endoscopic thyroidectomy using trans-axillary approach; surgical outcome of 581 patients. *Endocr J*. 2009;56(3):361–369.
5. Richmon JD, Pattani KM, Benhidjeb T, Tufano RP. Transoral robotic-assisted thyroidectomy: a preclinical feasibility study in 2 cadavers. *Head Neck*. 2011;33(3):330–333.
6. Anuwong A. Transoral endoscopic thyroidectomy vestibular approach: a series of the first 60 human cases. *World J Surg*. 2016;40(3):491–497.
7. Carta F, Mariani C, Marrosu V, Gerosa C, Puxeddu R. Three-dimensional, high-definition exoscopic parotidectomy: a valid alternative to magnified-assisted surgery. *Br J Oral Maxillofac Surg*. 2020;58(9):1128–1132.
8. Patel VA, Goyal N. Using a 4K-3D exoscope for upper airway stimulation surgery: proof-of-concept. *Ann Otol Rhinol Laryngol*. 2020;129(7):695–698.

CHAPTER

Exoscope application in free flap head and neck reconstruction

12

Armando De Virgilio, MD, PhD [1], Andrea Costantino, MD [2,3], Davide Di Santo, MD [3], Giuseppe Spriano, MD [4]

[1]*Assistant Professor of Otorhinolaryngology-Head and Neck Surgery, Humanitas University, Milan, Italy;* [2]*Department of Biomedical Sciences, Humanitas University, Pieve Emanuele, Milan, Italy;* [3]*Otorhinolaryngology Unit, IRCCS Humanitas Clinical and Research Center, Rozzano, Milan, Italy;* [4]*Professor and Chief of Otorhinolaryngology-Head and Neck Surgery, Humanitas University, Milan, Italy*

12.1 Introduction of 3D exoscopes in reconstructive microsurgery

Exoscopic technology was first introduced in free flap reconstruction in 2017. In particular, Piatkowski et al.[1] described their experience in breast reconstruction with a bilateral deep inferior epigastric perforator flap. The authors highlighted the lower depth of field compared to the operating microscope and the loss of resolution of the image at higher magnification. However, they believed in the potential of the exoscope in substituting the operating microscope with some adjustments in the future, especially underlying its versatility and ergonomic advantage.

During the last 2 years, several papers have been published reporting the feasibility of head and neck reconstruction using the exoscope. Ichikawa et al.[2] reported the use of the VITOM 3D exoscope in two cases for head and neck reconstruction with a free anterolateral thigh flap transfer. De Virgilio et al.[3] previously described the technical feasibility of microvascular anastomoses in 10 consecutive patients. The ORBEYE 3D exoscope (Olympus, Tokyo, Japan) was also used to perform three head and neck free flap reconstructions by Grammatica et al.[4] These papers allowed to better define the advantages and disadvantages of this system if compared to the operating microscope. Even if a direct comparison between these two systems is not available in the current literature, the exoscope demonstrated a high level of reliability and quality in terms of visualization and magnification of the surgical field.

The main application of the exoscope in head and neck free flap reconstruction is during the execution of microvascular anastomoses. However, the 3D vision and the modular magnification allow for augmented visualization also during free flap harvest and inset. The present chapter aims to provide a summary of the applications of the exoscopic technology to free flap head and neck reconstruction. In particular, the

Exoscope-Assisted Surgery in Otorhinolaryngology. https://doi.org/10.1016/B978-0-323-83168-0.00012-4

authors' experience is described to analyze the advantages and disadvantages of the exoscope in the execution of microvascular anastomoses.

12.2 Operating room set-up

As already mentioned in Chapter 1, the small size of the 3D camera and the slim holding system allow for a less cumbersome placement of the system if compared to the operating microscope. No interferences with the surgical field should be guaranteed during the procedure, and the main surgeon and the scrub nurse's movements should not be limited by the system. The exoscope is less cumbersome than the operating microscope, and it could be easily placed at the patient's feet during the microvascular anastomoses. As a consequence, the scrub nurse can position itself at the patient's head, without interfering with the screen visualization. The assistant surgeon can position itself next to, or in front of the main surgeon. However, in the latter case, a secondary screen should be placed for the assistant to achieve an adequate view of the surgical field. Other operating room (OR) members, such as students, should position themselves behind the main surgeon to maintain a perpendicular view of the screen. An example of the OR set-up during microvascular anastomoses is shown in Fig. 12.1.

If the operating exoscope is used during the free flap harvest, the OR set-up would be surely more complex. Free flap reconstruction is usually performed in the same timeframe by two different surgical teams, except for some centers. The exoscopic system could be easily placed at the patient feet if the free flap is taken from the lower extremities (e.g., fibula free flap or anterolateral thigh flap), while it is more difficult to find the right position during upper extremities free flap

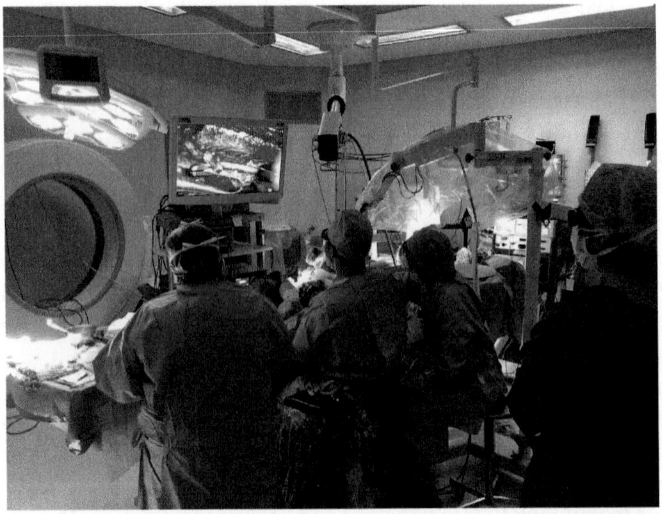

FIGURE 12.1

OR set-up during exoscope-assisted microvascular anastomosis.

harvesting (e.g., radial forearm free flap) without interfering with the head and neck tumor resection team.

12.3 Free flap harvest

Although an increased magnification is required to adequately perform a microvascular anastomoses due to the low diameter of vessels, the free flap harvest could be easily performed under direct vision. Surgical loupes are widely used to enhance the surgical field magnification, improving the ability to perform tissue dissection. Operating microscopes are rarely used to perform these surgical steps due to the high dimension of commonly used microscopes. On the other hand, the exoscope is less cumbersome than the operating microscope, and it could be used during free flap harvest as already mentioned earlier (Fig. 12.2).

Magnification of the surgical field could be particularly useful in the identification of septo-cutaneous and particularly myo-cutaneous perforators (Fig. 12.2B and C). Moreover, the 3D exoscope could be used to enhance the ability to perform precise dissection of fine structures avoiding damage to the vascular structures of the flap (Fig. 12.2A). Finally, it could reduce the donor site morbidity, allowing for the preservation of sensitive and motor nerve structures. The exoscope is extremely manageable and slim, so it can be prepared with sterile covers to be used only for crucial surgical steps. No additional costs and time is required from this perspective, given that the exoscope will be ready for the subsequent microvascular anastomoses.

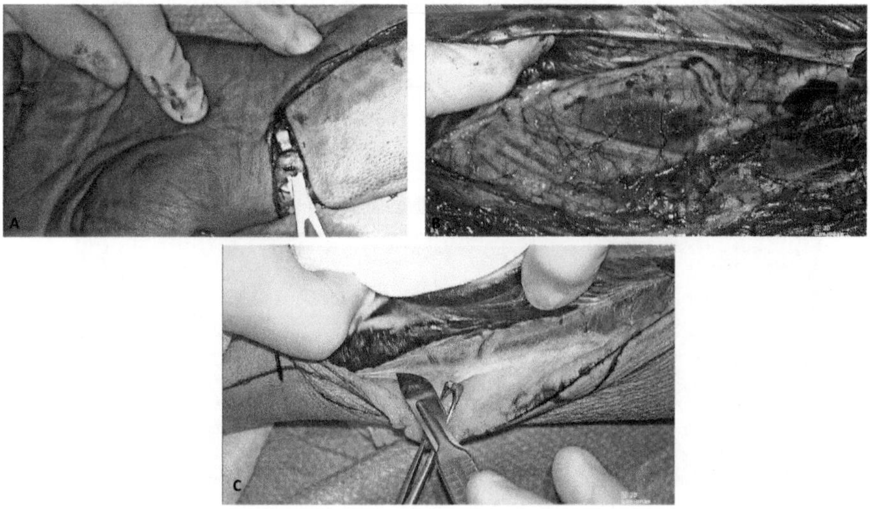

FIGURE 12.2

Exoscope-assisted free flap harvest of a radial forearm free flap (A), an anterolateral thigh free flap (B), and a fibula free flap (C).

12.4 Microvascular anastomoses

Microvascular anastomosis remains the most critical step in free tissue transfer, and approaches may vary among different centers. The ideal technique would cause the least trauma possible to the vessel wall, resulting in a reduction in the risk of thrombosis and an increase in short- and long-term patency rates. It is crucial to look for and isolate good quality vessels with a similar diameter. Another important aspect is to avoid any tension at the repair site and any stretches that could result in damage to the anastomosis. Moreover, it is essential to evert vessel walls while suturing to provide direct intima–intima contact.[5]

After the pedicle is ligated at the donor site, a partial flap inset is performed with or without the aid if the exoscope. Then, the holding system should be placed to obtain a focal distance of about 30 cm from the surgical field where the anastomoses should be performed. In our experience, this is the optimal distance to obtain an adequate working space to avoid any interferences during subtle maneuvering of the hands. The patient is placed in the Boyce position, with the neck rotated contralaterally and the sternocleidomastoid muscle retracted with self-retractors to improve the surgical field. The 3D exoscope is used to prepare both recipient and donor vessels. In particular, trimming of the adventitia is performed in the area of the proposed anastomosis and in the area where the clamp is to be applied. Background material (e.g., moist sponge) is placed beneath the vessel set-up, and vessel clamps are applied. Suturing technique is not different from the traditional one, and no limitations are determined by the use of the exoscope. Both end-to-end (Fig. 12.3) and

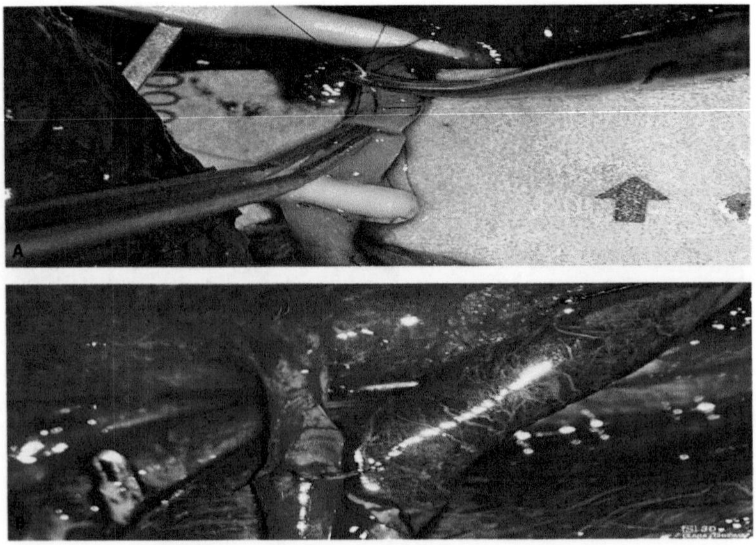

FIGURE 12.3

Exoscopic view of microvascular end-to-end arterial (A) and venous (B) anastomoses.

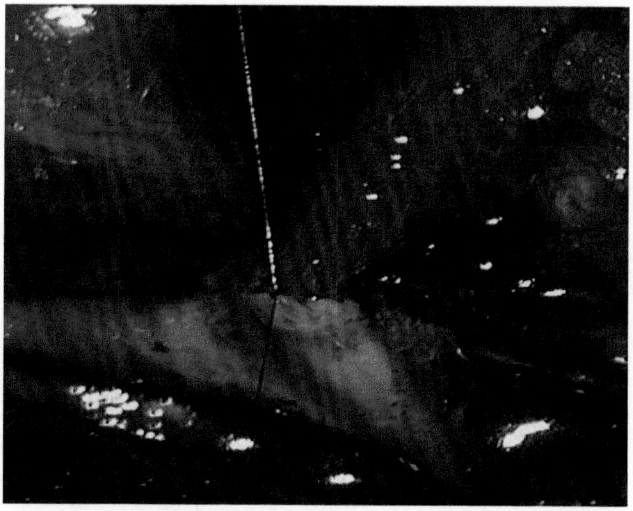

FIGURE 12.4

Exoscopic view of microvascular end-to-side venous anastomosis.

end-to-side (Fig. 12.4) anastomoses could be obviously performed. As a consequence, each surgeon could perform the anastomoses with its traditional technique.

12.5 Free flap inset

Free flap inset is a key step to achieve the adequate functional and aesthetic benefit in head and neck reconstruction. Several anatomical structures could need reconstruction in the head and neck area, and different skills and techniques should be applied to the specific case. Superficial reconstruction of the face and neck is commonly performed using local or regional flaps, while free flap reconstruction is usually needed to cover greater and deep defects. The flap inset is usually prepared before the microanastomoses to better define the pedicle length and orientation, other than to improve the stability of the vessels during the anastomoses. After the pedicle is attached to the recipient's vessels, the inset is completed to reconstruct the function and the appearance of the region.

The 3D exoscope could be used during these steps to enhance the surgical field magnification, particularly in deep areas such as the oral cavity (Fig. 12.5). These areas could be easily reached thanks to the great ergonomics of the exoscopic system. The 3D camera could be oriented in any direction during surgery, and it could be placed perpendicular to the surgical field. In addition, the image magnification could be modulated during surgery to focus anatomical structures of interest using the IMAGE1 PILOT. The importance of the educational role of the exoscope is clear during these steps. The exoscope could be used to share the surgical vision with

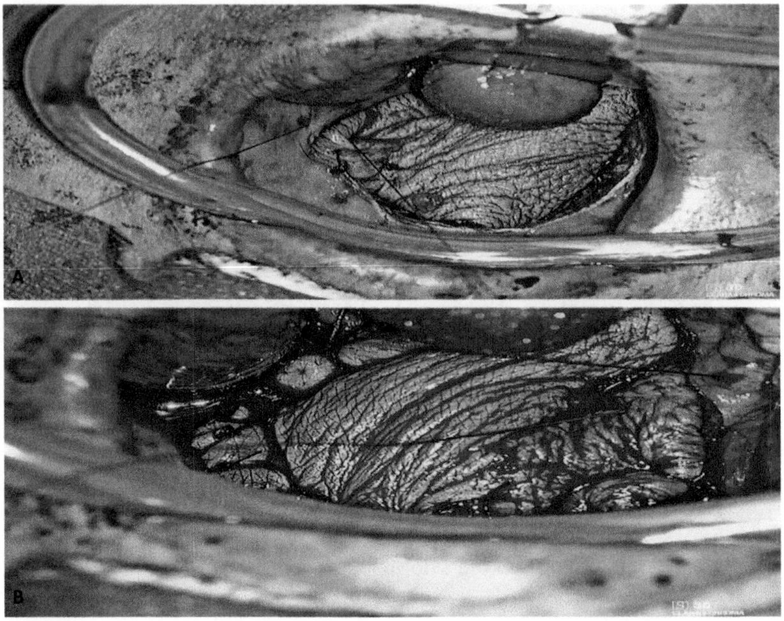

FIGURE 12.5

Radial forearm free flap inset for soft palate reconstruction after the resection of an adenoid cystic carcinoma.

other OR members that are rarely able to follow surgical steps in the oral cavity due to its depth. Moreover, the exoscope could be used to record the surgical steps for educational purposes.

12.6 Our experience

The VITOM 3D exoscope was used in our center for free flap head and neck reconstruction since April 2019. Thirty consecutive patients (males: 19; median age: 56.5, IQR: 44.7–66.5) have been treated to date. The exoscope was used for the microvascular anastomoses in all cases, while the free flap harvest and inset were performed with the exoscope only in a minority of patients ($n = 7$, 23.3%). All reconstructions have been performed using three different flaps. In particular, the anterolateral thigh free flap was the most used ($n = 13$, 43.3%). The fibula free flap was used in 11 (36.7%) cases that needed a bone reconstruction. Finally, the radial forearm free flap was chosen in only 6 (20%) cases. Different variants of the anterolateral thigh flap were used. In particular, it was harvested as fasciocutaneous ($n = 7$, 53.8%), myocutaneous ($n = 3$, 23.1%), and myofascial ($n = 3$, 23.1%) flap.

Reconstruction has been performed after primary tumor resection in all cases, and the majority of patients ($n = 22$, 73.3%) suffered from a head and neck squamous cell carcinoma. Tumors primary sites were as follows: oral cavity ($n = 21$, 70%), mandible ($n = 3$, 10%), orbital/eyelid ($n = 2$, 6.7%), maxilla ($n = 1$, 3.3%), paranasal sinuses ($n = 1$, 3.3%), ear ($n = 1$, 3.3%), and fronto-temporal area ($n = 1$, 3.3%).

The superior thyroid artery and the facial artery were prepared when possible in all cases before free flap arterial anastomosis. The thyro-linguo-facial venous trunk and its branches, and the external jugular vein were preserved when possible in all cases and prepared for a venous anastomosis. Then, the most suitable vessel was chosen for the anastomosis based on diameter matching. An adequate surgical view was acquired in all cases, and the microvascular anastomoses were performed successfully using the exoscope in all patients. The single end-to-end arterial anastomosis was performed in all cases. The median recipient artery diameter was 2.3 mm ($n = 30$, IQR: 1.8–2.6 mm), while the median donor artery diameter was 2.1 mm ($n = 30$, IQR: 2.0–2.8 mm). Venous anastomoses were end-to-end in 24 (80%) cases, while the internal jugular vein was used for an end-to-side anastomosis in 6 (20%) cases. In addition, a single venous anastomosis was performed in all cases. The median recipient vein diameter was 3.5 mm ($n = 24$, IQR 2.9–4.0 mm), while the median donor vein diameter was 3.0 mm ($n = 30$, IQR 2.8–3.5 mm).

The final free flap survival rate was 96.7%. Overall, the majority of patients ($n = 18$, 60%) did not develop any complications. The only free flap failure was observed in female patients who underwent tongue reconstruction with a forearm radial free flap after a squamous cell carcinoma resection. The other two patients experienced a free flap reconstruction-related complication. The venous anastomosis was revised in one patient due to a compressive neck hematoma on the second postoperative day. Another patient suffered from a deep infection of the donor site after a fibula frcc flap.

12.7 Advantages and disadvantages

12.7.1 A comparison with the operating microscope

The feasibility of microvascular anastomosis using the VITOM 3D exoscope in free flap head and neck reconstructive surgery is demonstrated by our case series. The operating microscope was not required during the anastomoses, and no complications were related to the reconstructive procedure.

The exoscope was developed to substitute the conventional surgical microscope in different procedures, and each kind of surgery requires specific characteristics to obtain the expected outcome.

We investigated the advantages and disadvantages of this surgical visualization and magnification tool to better understand the differences with the operating microscope in this specific clinical setting.

The VITOM 3D exoscope is controlled using an intuitive joystick through which the surgeon can adjust the video settings easily. The joystick is usually placed on the left of the main surgeon during the microvascular anastomoses. The surgeon can indeed modify the zoom and the focus easily during the procedure in complete autonomy. In particular, the image could be placed on the structures of interest without moving the camera. Only one hand is needed to adjust the video settings, as opposed to the operating microscope, enabling the surgeon to have a free hand able to maintain surgical instruments. As a consequence, the surgical procedure is surely faster and fluent avoiding the interruption inevitably encountered using the microscope.

Differences in terms of surgical setup were already mentioned earlier. This aspect should be underlined due to the potential impact on the clinical outcome. Some studies reported that the reduced dimension of the exoscope compared to the bulky operating microscope results in a wider surgical working space. Subtle maneuvering of the hands is required to perform the anastomoses, and no interferences or collisions with the camera should be encountered during the procedure. Moreover, easy manipulation of the instruments between the surgeon and the scrub nurse should be ensured to avoid any surgical delay or complication. In addition, the surgical discomfort is reduced during the anastomosis, improving the cervical spine health. The screen placed in front of the surgeon at eye level allows for a neutral cervical spine posture. The 3D camera could be horizontally oriented to reach deep areas during the anastomosis, while the surgeon could maintain an upright and neutral posture. Moreover, some areas could be difficultly reached using the microscope. For example, if the facial vessels are used to perform the microvascular anastomoses, an interposition of the mandibular bone could be encountered using the microscope. The anastomosis would be technically difficult with potential impairment of the postoperative outcome. Finally, the surgeon needs to maintain a fixed position for prolonged periods of time when using the binocular operating microscope, while the external screen used with the exoscope decouples the eyes from the microscope lens reducing the muscular tension at the cervical spine. On the other hand, the operating microscope gives a slightly better perception of depth and stereopsis by looking at the operating table through the eyepieces. This may result in a more direct and natural view thanks to the ability of physiologic eye accommodation, as well as the rounded field view that is wider than the rectangular one of the screen.

In the VITOM 3D exoscope, the combination of a 4K resolution with the 3D vision allows for adequate visualization of very fine details, such as a clot in the vessels lumen or signs of intimal tears. The magnifying power up to 30× is adequate for this procedure in the majority of cases as the diameter of vessels usually used in head and neck reconstruction is in the range of 1–3 mm. However, there are also some aspects worthy of improvement from this perspective. A loss of resolution is evident at higher magnification, particularly for vessels smaller than 1 mm. Even if no limitations were encountered in our experience, the loss of resolution could be a real disadvantage in supermicrosurgery.

Also the luminance provided by the exoscope could represent a limit during the anastomosis. The OR light should be maintained dimmed to obtain an adequate image quality on the high-definition screen. Moreover, the 3D glasses determine a darker vision that may cause difficulty for the scrub nurse in mounting the needles during the procedure. Finally, some nurses also complained about the eye strain due to the 3D video probably due to the partial distortion of the image when the gaze is not perfectly directed perpendicular to the screen. This results in a limitation especially to the assistant surgeon and scrub nurses if they are not perfectly in line with the sight of the main surgeon. However, a secondary screen could be used to overcome this issue as illustrated in Fig. 12.6.

The rectangular screen used during the procedure is set to a 16:9 format. As a consequence, the anastomoses are easily performed with a horizontal orientation. On the other hand, it could represent a relative disadvantage when performing anastomosis with a vertical orientation. This could force surgeons to perform undesired zoom-out maneuvers in some situations, such as end-to-side anastomosis, due to the limitation in the vertical extension of the surgical field (screen).

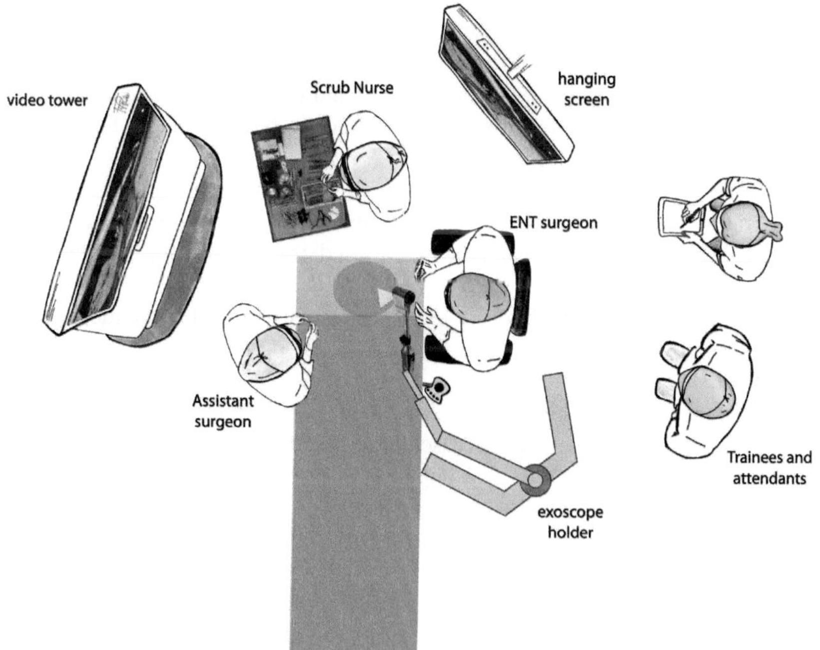

FIGURE 12.6

OR set-up example of exoscope-assisted microvascular anastomosis with two monitors.

12.8 Conclusions

The exoscope could be used to safely perform head and neck free flap reconstructive procedures, and it represents a valuable alternative to the surgical microscope in reconstructive microsurgery. The analysis of the pros and cons of the exoscope implies a comparison with the operating microscope. The ergonomics, the ease of using, and the possibility to share the view among all the OR members represent the main advantages of this system. We should bear in mind that exoscopic technology was recently introduced in the clinical practice, and only a few centers have a long-lasting experience with this tool, particularly for free flap reconstruction. However, this promising technology is becoming more and more widespread in several specialties and centers. Further technical improvements are expected in the near future to improve some technical aspects, such as the relatively low luminance and the eye strain determined by the 3D glasses.

12.9 Pearls and pitfalls

- The exoscope could be used to safely perform head and neck free flap reconstructive procedures, and it represents a valuable alternative to the surgical microscope in reconstructive microsurgery.
- The main application of the exoscope in head and neck free flap reconstruction is during the execution of microvascular anastomoses, but it could be helpful also during free flap harvest and inset.
- The ergonomics, the ease of use, and the possibility to share the view among all the operating room members represent the main advantages of this system.
- The relatively low luminance and the eye strain determined by the 3D glasses can still be improved.
- Magnification of the surgical field could be particularly useful in the identification of septo-cutaneous and particularly myo-cutaneous perforators during free flap harvest.
- The exoscope could enhance the ability to perform precise dissection of fine structures avoiding damage to the vascular structures of the flap.
- The exoscope could be used for free flap inset in deep areas, such as the oral cavity.

References

1. Piatkowski AA, Keuter XHA, Schols RM, van der Hulst RRWJ. Potential of performing a microvascular free flap reconstruction using solely a 3D exoscope instead of a conventional microscope. *J Plast Reconstr Aesthet Surg*. 2018;71(11):1664–1678.
2. Ichikawa Y, Senda D, Shingyochi Y, Mizuno H. Potential advantages of using three-dimensional exoscope for microvascular anastomosis in free flap transfer. *Plast Reconstr Surg*. 2019;144(4):726e–727e.

3. De Virgilio A, Iocca O, Di Maio P, et al. Free flap microvascular anastomosis in head and neck reconstruction using a 4K three-dimensional exoscope system (VITOM 3D). *Int J Oral Maxillofac Surg*. 2020;49(9):1169−1173.
4. Grammatica A, Schreiber A, Vural A, et al. Application of a 3D 4K exoscopic system to head and neck reconstruction: a feasibility study. *Eur J Plast Surg*. 2019;42(6):611−614.
5. Wei F, Mardini F. *Flaps and Reconstructive Surgery*. 2nd ed. Amsterdam: Elsevier; 2017.

Further reading

1. Cheng H-T, Ma H, Tsai C-H, Hsu W-L, Wang T-H. A three-dimensional stereoscopic monitor system in microscopic vascular anastomosis. *Microsurgery*. 2012;32(7): 571−574.

Index

'*Note*: Page numbers followed by "f" indicate figures.'

R

S

T

V

W

X

Printed and bound by CPI Group (UK) Ltd, Croydon, CR0 4YY
08/05/2025
01864763-0002